MILESTONES IN MEDICINE

Milestones in Medicine

Laity Lectures of the New York Academy of Medicine

Introduction by

JAMES ALEXANDER MILLER, M.D.
PRESIDENT, NEW YORK ACADEMY OF MEDICINE

Essay Index Reprint Series

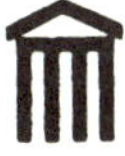

BOOKS FOR LIBRARIES PRESS
FREEPORT, NEW YORK

Reprinted 1971 by arrangement with
Hawthorn Books, Inc.

INTERNATIONAL STANDARD BOOK NUMBER:
0-8369-2119-4

LIBRARY OF CONGRESS CATALOG CARD NUMBER:
73-142681

PRINTED IN THE UNITED STATES OF AMERICA

INTRODUCTION

THE enthusiasm with which the public responded to the first series of laity lectures, prompted the New York Academy of Medicine to continue this educational service. The lectures of the 1936-37 series are published herein, and are thus made available to an audience much greater than that housed in Hosack Hall.

There is gratification in the success of the laity lectures. For thus the ventured judgment of those who initiated this service has been validated. In their opinion the public wishes not only to know but also to understand.

There is a substantial difference between knowing and understanding. To know, is to have acquaintance with, to recognize, while to understand is to appreciate the meaning and import of what is known. The act of understanding thus presupposes knowledge and makes critical judgment possible.

Knowledge alone is an inadequate basis upon which to found judgment: in medicine perhaps more so than in any other branch of science. For example, it is common knowledge that the rhythmic contractions of the heart produce electrical currents and that these currents may be registered by means of an electrical apparatus known as electrocardiograph. It is thus possible to diagnose certain changes in heart structure and function by a study of the electrical currents produced by the heart. This is called electrodiagnosis. Many knowing of this feat of modern medicine, precisely because of this knowledge, have fallen victims to unscrupulous quacks, who pretend that they can electrodiagnose all diseases to which the human flesh is heir, from anemia to zoster.

Knowledge of the initial fact makes the expectation of universal electrodiagnosis "reasonable." Understanding, however, at once dispels this expectation. Similarly an understanding of endocrines and of vitamins exposes thoroughly the spurious claims of those who incorporate them in a variety of cosmetics, and vend them as skin rejuvenators, fountains of youth, and the like.

The laity lectures of the New York Academy of Medicine are unique in that by an historical presentation of the development of medicine's ideologies, knowledge and techniques, not only the established facts are presented, but also the sequence of and reasons for their evolution. Thus understanding as well as knowledge is promoted.

No less gratifying than the enthusiastic response of the public has been the generous coöperation of the lecturers. They have taken time and energy in the midst of their appointed and pressing labors, to tell the story of medicine, in its broad implications, or from the more restricted but elaborated viewpoint of the specialist.

To them, especially, the Academy is indebted for their aid in maintaining and furthering the best traditions of medicine.

JAMES ALEXANDER MILLER, M.D.
President, The New York Academy of Medicine

CONTENTS

I

THE HISTORICAL BACKGROUND OF PSYCHIATRY

BY

SMITH ELY JELLIFFE, M.D.

I

THE HISTORICAL BACKGROUND OF PSYCHIATRY

History—background—psychiatry: An ambitious, enticing and yet at the same time a perplexing program. Where shall we begin?

Old Man River has many sources of origin as a completed happening. It just goes "rollin' along," but has had many starting places. Perhaps we can best begin our story with the subject matter. "In the beginning was the word"—*Psychiatry.* And so to the dictionaries; manifestly first to the Greek.

Here our initial clue comes through the word ψυχή, Psyche. What did it stand for in the historical past? How far back can we trace its origins without too great an exercise of philological erudition? What changes has it undergone and, at the present time, what may it have accumulated as to meaning and significance?

If we should ask the first man in the street the meaning of psyche, the answer—if one received any at all—probably would be "mind"; and so, in a sense, did the word also mean mind for the Greeks, but only in a very limited way. The Greeks were nearer to certain realities than the man in the street of to-day.

From the times of Homer to the beginning of the

Christian era there was a history of about a thousand years. We shall not attempt to traverse it with the philologists, but we will take a glance at some of the Homeric meanings: mind, and other more important ones.

The word counters have told us that in the *Iliad* ψυχή appears thirty-five, and in the *Odyssey* forty-two times. Meaning what?

In a dynamic, acting, doing, living world verbal connotations preceded nouns and thus it is proper to find the noun ψυχή derived from the verb ψυχω, to breathe. For the earliest observers, all the higher animals breathed, but only when alive. When they died they ceased breathing and where, arose the query, did the breathing go? It was and then was not, and even in prehistory was bound up in life and death. Something left the body and at the moment of death. It was chiefly on this aspect that the Homeric poems dwelt, and certain philologists tell us it represented for Homer the animal and not the spiritual life.

But what of the innumerable acts of breathing during life? Did the Homeric poems make any distinction between these breathings and the last breath when something left the body? Further, the ψυχή left the body in other ways than the breath for the ancients. If one recalls the story of Sarpedon we note that the lance of Patroclus struck him in the center of the chest and he fell like a gigantic tree stricken in the forest. He implored his friend Glaucus to assemble the Lycians to save his body, but Patroclus, wrenching free his lance, his ψχυή escaped by way of the wounds. It was something volatile, cold, subterranean, and came from Hades to which it returned. In the Homeric poems it was compared to the smoke that disappeared, or was like a feeble noise in the earth that had vanished.

In the *Odyssey* (XI, 219-222), Ulysses at the time of his visit to his mother in Hades learned from her something about the ψυχή. In Murray's translation it reads, "For the sinews no longer hold the flesh and the bones together, but the strong might of blazing fire destroys these, as soon as life leaves the white bones, and the spirit, like a dream, flits away, and hovers to and fro."

I am no Greek scholar, and this little parade of learning is all borrowed but, still pilfering from reliable sources, let us see what happens to this ψυχή, this spirit, which must rejoin something in Hades, and around which the ritual of cremation was so involved. A ritual be it recalled stemming from paleolithic times. The ψυχή had some standing. There were the best circles in Hades to be entered and by the appropriate cremation ceremonials if, with Justesen,[1] the ψυχή was not to be thrown to the dogs of which there were plenty in the lower regions, then as now.

Before burning, however, the ψυχή may not have left the body entirely on its trip to Hades. Thus in the condition of fainting it hovered about ready to return when consciousness was regained. In the *Odyssey* (XXIV, 347-348), Laertes thinks this is true when

[1] Justesen. *Les principes psychologiques d'Homere* (Copenhagen, 1928).

his son fainted. In the Homeric view, the ψυχή, during sleep, remained within the body, passive and receptive.

It would take us too far from the immediate interest of our subject were we to go much further with Homer and his conceptions of the ψυχή. There is one conception, however, which must not be overlooked, since therein we may see, by a slight refocusing, how modern Homer was.

In one place in the *Odyssey* (XI, 45), we read how the ψυχή loves the taste of blood. It is significant that Homer attaches a mental attribute to blood much as, to anticipate a bit, the psychoanalyst claims that the energy of the libido may be invested in blood, or the blood-making organs, or any and all organs of the body. It is not my intention to homologize the libido of Freud with the ψυχή of Homer, but we may find some more than superficial resemblances.

Inasmuch as these ancients and even their paleolithic ancestors cremated a part of a loved animal with the dead this, as well as other evidence, points to the fact that the ψυχή was to be found in lower animals as well. The comparative psychologist of today, testifies in a definitely Homeric strain.

Of the later Greeks, Hesiod is said not to have used the word. In Anacreon we find an interesting gloss. Here ψυχή corresponds to Soul; also it is the equivalent of Character, of Disposition. Again we find it signifying Conscience and in one place it means the Me, My. Pindar has it as "astral body," as "life," as "soul," and the ψυχ'χί after being banished for their sins become purified and return to the earth reincarnated as saintly heroes.

As for Æschylus, Sophocles and Euripides, those ancient Greek tragedians whom Whitehead[2] has ingeniously declared were the "Pilgrim Fathers of the modern scientific imagination," Justesen has industriously gathered the meanings they gave to the ψυχή which he finds used in one hundred and twenty-five passages. Eight times it is used as "Astral Body," forty-eight times signifying "Life," thirty-six times as "Soul," twenty-five as the "Me," and twelve as the "Individual," "the Person."

Let us go with the majority and thus come to a general conclusion that ψυχή and "Life" are one. It is the Me, the "Life Principle" working within the body and thus most aptly is the subject matter of psychiatry. Here among the Greeks there is little cavil that the individual as a whole is a well-documented principle.

It will be apparent that I have taken the liberty of departing very far from what I believe most of you have expected. On first thought I apprehend that my title evoked in most of you at least a vision of something quite different from Greek roots. I am certain that ideas of Bedlam, Bloomingdale, of State Hospitals, of the insane asylums, of the battles in courtrooms over wills, or responsibility for homicidal acts, and so on, were closer to your consciousness and more significant than the glosses from Homer or Pindar or Sophocles. I promise however not to entirely disap-

2 Whitehead, *Science and the Modern World* (New York, 1932).

point those with such preconceptions, but it is my purpose to indicate that psychiatry is a far wider and deeper discipline than merely that which is confined to social instruments circumscribing the lives of all too many of us, or concerned with the antics and phantasies of the mentally ill.

Psychiatry in the sense in which I wish to present it is the oldest of the medical arts. I have called it the "fairy godmother of medicine," Dr. J. Ramsay Hunt more aptly the "Queen Mother of Medicine." Under innumerable forms psychiatry has been practised from the earliest times. The ancient Greeks, as I have briefly indicated sought, for example, in the one ceremonial alone—that of cremation—to lead the ψυχ'χί to a better standing in Hades.

The Hades of modern times is as ominous as any of the past. It is not something tucked away in a cavern. It is with us all the time. It exists in the innumerable forms of human slavery: of dishonest and corrupt social institutions. It is found not alone in the distraught mental field but many chronic irreversible bodily diseases may aptly and correctly be termed organ psychoses. It is the function of modern-day psychiatry to enter into these recesses of Hades and obtain for the ψυχ'χί better standing. To give them face. To free them for creative action.

Let us now pass to another historical background in our quest for understanding of the entire psyche. What is this ψυχή, this Me, this that was and is not? This life that leaves behind it dead matter? This entropy of energy which has run down to a definition of "space and time"? For if I am not very much mistaken we must say a word about matter, and the ψυχή in matter, much as the Greeks spoke of it in blood, in the lower animals, and in everything.

Ions, elements, chemical affinities, enzymes, hormones, cells, organs, bodies, me, you, society! What has been the march in these advancing organizations? I doubt if it will serve our purpose to delve too deeply into this advancing synthesis which time has brought into experimental something. Eons and eons of time!

You may smile—I did—when first I read in a highly prized work on biochemistry of the "psychology of nitrogen." In this conception not only does nitrogen have a ψυχή but so also does phosphorus and calcium and oxygen and the rest of the ninety-two elements. As I skirt around the edge and peer into the depths of the Vesuvian crater of the chemical past of matter a ribald epitaph warns me to beware. It reads:

Here lies the body of Robert Gordon
  Mouth almighty and teeth accordin
Stranger tread lightly o'er this wonder
  If he opens his mouth your gone by thunder.

So I shall step very lightly over the ψυχή of the chemical elements. But they are there, so don't be misled.

In fact, whenever we get on the constantly developing road of psychiatry we may be surprised to learn of the number of spirits that the primitive man projected into the Cosmos about him and those that modern man still projects though not so conspicuously in their ancient form. So far as average experience goes some of these projections are only known to those who have some experience with delirium tremens. In that condition one may see the ancient spirit world in its accompanying infantile fears chiefly related to animal identifications. A study of this animal world is full of interest, but we shall defer it.

Before we return to our more explicit path let me fragmentarily indicate how through the centuries man has sought the ψυχή in the chemistry of the body. We have read much of the philosopher's stone. For the hoi polloi it was a stone that would turn base metal into gold. This was the vulgar conception, and we read of the alchemists of medieval days, and much of the transmutation of metals. The more profound scholar, however, was not interested in such childish activities. For such the making of something higher was the search for the life principle, and in the crucibles of many an alchemist's laboratory the search was to produce life, the homunculus, and further, we are certain that much of that which we call the higher spiritual life was involved in the quest. Sublimation was the word they used then when working with the subtle metal mercury, and sublimation is the word we use now when speaking of the putting of our sexual energy to higher social aims. Much as when the Greeks were afraid to lose face when they were to go to Hades, modern man seeks social approval by the process of sublimation.

Rapidly flying through the ages to the present time we see a host of busy workers exploiting the chemical ψυχή in their efforts to solve psychiatric problems. One could touch lightly on the use of mercury and include its close family relatives, arsenic and bismuth, as devil chasers. Mercury we are told was used by the Chinese several thousand years ago as a reconstructive agent. As cinnabar it was not used for the treatment of syphilis either by the Chinese or by the native American Indian of the stone age in their vapor baths. Here again it was used as a reconstructive agent, a sublimation process. *Steam,* then, as now, undoubtedly contributed to the reconstruction of the body since steam was also breath; ψυχή, the Soul, that rose out of the water just as the breath congealed, was seen by the ancients as a corporeal body. Hence the Ghost.

Our modern biochemically inclined epileptologists, going back to Hippocrates, might be glanced at as we hurry by. Hippocrates wrote, "But whoever is acquainted with such a change in man and can render a man humid and dry, hot and cold by regimen could also cure his disease without minding purifications, spells and all other illiberal practices of a like kind." Only within the last few years, quite naïvely state some of these physicians, has the truth of Hippocrates's thought been demonstrated. Paralleling his concept but paraphrasing his words, they write, "we may say that whoever is acquainted with physiology and can render a man non-acidotic, dehydrated, and fully oxygenated could also repress his disease without purification of narcissistic personalities, ritualistic empirical diets and all other practices of a like kind.

Thus may I be privileged to insist we find a looking towards the alchemistic patterning. Take out the acids, reduce the water and increase the oxygen, and the Herculean furor is to be banished.

Certainly cremation did all of this but our Greeks knew there were other than chemical elements in the body. They knew that something escaped, and we have seen somewhat of its reception in Hades, if the so-called "illiberal practices" of some of our moderns had been correctly carried out.

And so without much further ado let us take up again the trail of the ψυχή when life insinuated itself into dead matter, as Bergson puts it.

I would like to discuss briefly the spirit of the Dryad and related myths which deal with the ψυχή in other terms; spirits, gnomes, elfs, devils, and the host of synonymous dwellers within the body.

In order to give this array of uncanny creations a concrete setting and still keeping in mind the chemical background, let me offer myself as an experimental guinea-pig and glimpse one or more of my annoyances, my *Agrimonia fastidiosæ,* as Dr. Dana so frequently quoted Horace as authority. It touches upon the mysterious and dark chemical background suggested by the acidotic, dehydrated dummy of the chemical thinking epileptologists.

Some few years back I began to notice that when a door slammed, I jumped. When the telephone bell rang beside me while quietly reading or writing I was startled. So most of you have responded, but *my* jump, *my* startle was exaggerated. When I am sitting quietly if something brushes against my leg it jerks. The kick is also exaggerated. Further I notice with increasing annoyance that I will suddenly turn my head or start to glimpse what seems something or somebody at my side or behind me to realize almost at the same instant that it is but the glint of something on my glasses, or perhaps a straggling hair of my eyebrow. Even more and, now with amusement, I apprehend the presence of a person in uniform strikingly resembling a bell-hop, or one of the doormen so beautifully uniformed as on Park Avenue, or even a policeman, only to find that it is but an illusion created by a stack of box-like drawers in my secretary's office which passing from my reception room to my office I would note several times a day, each drawer with its small white label, into which I distribute reprints classified and in order. The upright row of labels is sufficient to cause a faulty identification with the row of buttons of the projected uniform.

Here is something to be thought about, not to be feared, since my reality tester, my Ego, in the Freudian sense, instantaneously resolves the buttons into the reprint classifying labels on my stack of drawers. The Me, the person, however, behind all this had been startled, had turned, had kicked, had momentarily made something real into something unreal. What was it—this almost convulsive starting, this illusional seeing and believing?

This sensitiveness, or vigilance, had on closer examination more technical attendant signs. I—your guinea-pig—showed notably increased knee, elbow and wrist jerks and a group of small signs or symptoms which the neurologist would recognize as something akin to the disorder known as spasmophilia or even tetany. If still more exaggerated this condition might permit the escape of a more volcanic reaction, such as a convulsive discharge. Your guinea-pig might have fits. Were it not for some degree of nerve deafness it is not impossible that the hearing machinery might show a similar tendency to falsification and that auditory illusions might have to be corrected like the others. You all know how suspicious deaf people are said to be.

In brief the solid, heavy, deliberate, and stocky guinea-pig, the writer, while not exactly a Hamlet, assailed and tormented by the slings and arrows of outrageous fortune, conceals a more susceptible, more sensitive, more vigilant body ready to respond at the drop of the hat to very slight and insignificant stimuli.

Reduced to a simple formula, the importance of which has already been touched upon, there is something going on in the nature of a conflict between the realities of the Cosmic forces and the Ego. Using my earlier terms ψυχή, the dryads, the spirits, the devils, known even in Homeric times to be resident in the blood and in all of the organs of the body, are seeking some form of escape, some expression in action. The start, the kick, the turning of the head, the illusion of the bell-hop, these are minor forms of the Dryads effort to be released, held by the forces of rational intelligence, that is by the defense functions of the Ego.

This may all be very interesting but where are the ideas concerning the background of psychiatry? It may be my reader apprehends that I am slowly closing in on the central theme of this discussion. The technic is an old one, roughly recalling Browning's *Ring and the Book* or the simple device of the geographer who would trace each headwater in following the development of a river.

And so permit me to cross my track and double on the hypervigilance this time with an eye again to the chemical background. Here your guinea-pig must tell more about himself to reveal what lies behind this hypervigilance. The chief situation which I would reveal is a certain method of talking and of breathing while talking. In brief it consists in an exaggerated effort to get as many words out of each breath as possible. Each expiration must be squeezed to the last gurgle. Thus there results a deep inspiration and then this push, not necessarily a rush, to deliver as much as possible even to the last gasp. It became a habit not particularly noticeable, except now and then, to an acute observer. I do not run down like the wobble of a gramophone record. I shall not go into further details how this mechanism had a lot of ingenious imitators in other acts and anticipated acts of the body. These continued for years. Inasmuch as at times there was a lot of talking in discussion or exposition this hyperventilation of the lungs was constant. There was much-too-much air conditioning in my make-up.

What this hyperventilation means involves us again in the physiological background. There is as most people know a certain amount of residual carbon dioxide in the lung alveoli while we are breathing. It acts as a sort of buffer, or cushion in the oxidizing process in order that the alkali of the blood will not be called upon too rapidly to neutralize the acidifying process of oxygenation. Thus we keep on the alkali side. If inspiration and expiration are exaggerated, that is, if there is hyperventilation, the alkalies of the body are heavily drawn upon in order to counteract acidosis. The alkali that is chiefly used is calcium. With too great a hyperventilation the alkali reserve runs down and a diminished calcemia develops. This hypocalcemia lies behind the condition known as tetany and so we are approaching my start, my kick, my illusory policeman. For calcium is a very important element in the wiring up of the nervous system. Briefly this nervous system of ours is a vast switchboard with incoming and outgoing bits of apparatus all working on cells and wires which are arranged end to end with short gaps at each junction. Here two membranes touch each other. This is the neuron theory. At each juncture there is an electrical resistance that serves to prevent impulses from passing over too easily. Calcium keeps up this resistance at the synaptic junction. With hypocalcemia the membrane is more vulnerable and both the incoming and outgoing calls go through the switchboard too intensely. Here is a part of the explanation of the hypersensitivity of your guinea-pig. The biochemist or the physiologist is usually content to leave the problem here. He may possibly go on to question the parathyroid gland, since this gland is thought to mobilize calcium or to aid in its distribution. We shall also take a glimpse at the bones where reserves of calcium are stored for daily use and for emergencies.

A picture of the skull bones of your experimental guinea-pig, if it were possible to show one, would reveal that my hyperventilation has called upon its calcium supply heavily. It has dug pockets into it so that the X-ray experts speak of the skull as a Paget skull. I have mentioned previously the fact that the biochemist, the physiologist and, yes, even the endocrinologist, abandon their quest at the calcium level, the synaptic junction level, or the parathyroid level. They are all involved but the answer is not yet without the look in of the psychiatrist who demands to know what your guinea-pig's ψυχή has been trying to do with this breathing foolishness. What is the ψυχή getting out of this habitual form of speech or even thinking, or other fundamentally related type of effort?

In order to learn of this breathing behavior we must go back to another source in the background. This time to the psychology of infancy. I have told you that the most outstanding feature of this hyperventilation was the squeezing effort to get all the words possible out of each breath. I have pointed out the possibilities of excessive exposition and were it not that at times I am mute, and these are protracted, I had been gathered to my fathers long ere this.

Childhood is, after all, a long way on the journey in the waters of life. Our vision of the earlier springs and brooks of the infantile phases of the psyche that precede childhood is as yet very hazy. I have intimated something of this in the suggestion regarding the ψυχή of inorganic matter. Of the fetal ψυχή we can but state more or less generally accepted biological principles. One of these is the principle of recapitulation which in its simplest form states that the fetus goes through the various stages of life that have preceded it in the evolutionary scale. Dr. Foster Kennedy illustrated certain features of this.[3] If we accept the findings of geologists certain forms of bacterial life were present on this earth at least two to three billion years ago. Even supposing it were a few hundred million years, certainly this is enough to make us pause as to the experience locked up in the ψυχή of the present-date human fetus. We may contemplate this mystery in the comic form of my quoted epitaph of Mr. Robert Gordon or we may sink into a mystic participation of the past and phrase it as one of the glories of God. No matter how you look at it the psyche or life principle is traveling fast in its fetal journey. How fast I would not venture to conjecture. Light, the physicist tells us, is traveling at about one hundred and eighty-six thousand miles a

[3] Foster Kennedy, "The Organic Background of Mind," *Medicine and Mankind* (New York, 1936).

second. I suspect that the psyche of the fetus has hitched its wagon to a star and is going along quite as fast in its two hundred and eighty day traversing of the billion years of recapitulation of experience. I am certain that environment and the ψυχή are at it hammer and tongs all through this period. There is a continuous bipolar conflict between restraint and freedom; the Hegelian synthesis, let us surmise, being resolved in the forward thrust of development. How much squeezing takes place and is evidenced in the kicking fetus of five to six months I do not know. How much the lung ψυχή wishes to leave its amphibian intrauterine adaptation for the greater freedom of the air-earned animal I have only the empty words to query. We do know, however, that the process of birth is accomplished in one mighty squeeze. Whether my own was great or small history telleth not. I was number four in the family procession so that being the first to suffer the trauma of birth cannot be my alibi. I must look in other directions for light on the squeeze. I do know that throughout adolescence a familiar dream was of "passing through a city in a canal," possibly a birth dream, but to my recollection there was never any anxiety about the dream. It was always a pleasant trip on a canal-boat and probably had some other connotation. More probably some bladder displacement and recompense. Psychiatric backgrounds begin to be clearer in the new functions of nursing, of urination and of defecation, for here there is holding and possessing, rejection and losing. Here the observant mother may learn much of the child's utilization of the ψυχή, for this is the golden era of character formation. The patterns of later performance such as the breathing I have spoken of are beginning to be laid down. Biologists call these patterns, Aristotle spoke of them as ends or entelechies, the Greeks spoke of them as Fate. The church uses the phrase God's Will.

An ancient wise man, Protagoras, said that for the ordinary man the phrasing was indifferent. It was not his business to query why. The aspect, or ideology, with which the individual could get along best was perhaps the wisest. For the man of exact measurement, however, for those who still battle to gain control over the reality of the environment, that is, the scientist, he must phrase it more precisely if new regions of the Cosmos are to come under the Promethean desire to steal the ψυχή from inorganic matter and the hidden forces of the world about us.

It was the acme of wisdom for that colored sergeant, who during the war told his squad that T.N.T. meant, "Travel, nigger, travel," but the skilled chemist knew that that was but one aspect of reality hiding behind a chemical symbol.

If I am to get any nearer the significance of the squeezing pattern of your guinea-pig, which in the formula that starts with "this is the maiden all forlorn," that caused the breathing habit, that produced the hyperventilation, that threatened the acid base equilibrium, that robbed the bones and wasted the calcium, that overburdened the parathyroid and all to be behind the sudden kick, the turning of the head, the illusion of the bell-hop, I cannot be satisfied with the man in the street's interpretation that I am "oversensitive." The psychiatrist who is desirous of controlling the demon in the ψυχή must go through from the "maiden all forlorn" to "house that Jack built," if he is to get anywhere. Fortunate is any man who can grasp all of the stages in any complicated life process, especially when it deals with some even slight anomaly of behavior, such as the knocking on wood, or the use of amber beads, or wearing a hair shirt, or not lighting three cigarettes with one match, or living on the thirteenth floor, or a thousand, yes, tens of thousands of minor peccadillos of mankind's curious and interesting compulsions and beliefs occurring in his everyday behavior.

I shall not dissect your guinea-pig any further. I shall simply state that some portion of the factor of infantile grasping, of squeezing, of desire and need to master the bladder, the intestine, muscular control for reasons as yet unfathomed, had been displaced to the language apparatus and there worked havoc with the best interests of the individual.

What I wish to emphasize is that the psychiatric background is the most important part of the picture if understanding is to be reached. The chemical ψυχή is there, the physiological ψυχή is there, but without a glimpse of what motivation is behind the combined φυχχί real wisdom has not been achieved.

There are innumerable situations in life where the sergeant's admonition to "travel, nigger, travel" is of much greater value than the minute analysis of complex situations. Happy are those who can arrive at a simple grasp of reality, intuitional if you will, rather than being hindered by the uncertainties arising from the conflict of opinions. I regret I cannot speak, in this brief discussion, of the tyranny of vested ideologies, under the head of the mental institution of the Super-Ego, and its complicity in the actual aiding, abetting or definitely causing a brain, liver, kidney, or lung psychosis.

So again by going back to another starting place of our background we come to that fountainhead, that deals more intimately at least to the lay mind with the mental illnesses, the psychoses.

It is not my intention to offer you a history of psychiatry. This is too technical a subject and one of comparatively little interest outside of the professional ranks. But I do wish to be a bit more precise about the definition of a psychosis which is the starting point of a more explicit consideration of the main framework of psychiatry.

I shall offer as a guide the Freudian conception of the psychotic mechanism. I have hinted at it all along, or rather been laying the foundations. In brief it is a conflict between the Ego and reality in which the Ego must give way to the satisfaction of instinctual cravings through a distortion of reality. The Ego, in the psychiatric sense in which I use it, is chiefly that mental institution that tests reality. In popular parlance we can speak of it as reason, as intelligence, as partly intuitional. I do not mean by the Ego what is usually understood by it, namely, the egotistical

Me. The word is used in a variety of ways but here we use it as a tester of reality, such as when your guinea-pig realized that there was no bell-hop, there were no people behind him. My Ego quickly recognized the labels as labels; the glint on the glasses. But you can readily note that the guinea-pig was walking on a very narrow edge. If his Ego had not stood up we would be in the psychiatric kingdom of phantasy. Were your guinea-pig to have exclaimed as he passed by the apparition of the neatly labeled reprint boxes, "Here boy, send up a bottle of vichy and two glasses to room 55," he surely would have passed over into the psychotic world, and Hades, instead of remaining in his background, would have been right there and not far from the Bellevue Psychiatric Hospital.

And now to another bit of the background. Once I took a walking trip through Switzerland. It was during my *Wanderjahr.* It included coming down the valley of the Rhône. One of the outstanding memories was the sight of the Rhône river-water, glacial colored as it extended far out into Lake Geneva, showing in strong contrast to the more settled clear waters on each side of it. It stretched miles before its waters were merged with those of the larger body.

Some such analogy is to be seen in our study. It refers to certain muddy waters which merge with those of our psychiatric body of ideas. They come from an ancient source, coeval with the head-waters of the ψυχή. The reader will recall that, at one time in the history of social organization, lawyer, priest, and doctor were combined in the person of the early medicine man. The turbid stream—I use the term in no derogatory meaning—is the legal one.

It was inevitable that as soon as property and tools accumulated there was strife, and society had to specialize. The lawyer became the mediator. I am only thumb-sketching and may be caricaturing but I wish to call attention to a very interesting difference in the cultural life of the Greeks and the Romans which bears on our background.

When problems of anomalous and variable behavior arose which were sufficiently great or inconvenient to the body politic, the Greek analyzed the ψυχή and devised methods of treatment. They were subtle and ingenious and the whole body of Greek thought constitutes the present world's most precious possession. In fact some men of learning have said that everything of value in present-day cultural thought had its origin in Greece.

When Rome conquered the Western world the aggressive-possessive cravings of the human animal entered largely into his cultural patterns. When it came to the discussion of mental disorders in those earlier days the Romans were impatient with what they termed Greek subtleties. Possibly they were incapable of understanding them—a not uncommon method of defense. So in a manner of speaking, they said, and chiefly when property rights were under discussion, away with these analytical, hair-splitting intricacies of the Greeks; their paranoias, their amentias, their hypochondrias and other terms of differentiation of mental diseases as we would call them to-day. We will lump them all together and call them *insaniens*. Hence arose from a complex generalization the word "insanity." Its stupidities still cling to it and chiefly in that muddy stream of thinking used by the lawyers to the present day. Side by side with the concept of mental disease there has run this legal monstrosity, "insanity," and few there are who can separate the concepts. Thus we hear the asinine statement "medically insane but legally sane." I will dwell briefly on this unfortunate situation since it belongs in both background and foreground of psychiatry.

"Insanity" is not a medical concept and has no place in psychiatry proper. It should have only legal connotations. In short, and the phraseology in law is often quite accurate, "insanity" is a social status. Only Courts of Law can make insanity. It does so in relation to certain definite issues, and there are at least a dozen of them, all according to definitions which vary more or less in the forty-eight different states of the Union. These all follow a fairly uniform pattern which states that if a person who is to have his social responsibility tested, if he has a mental disorder or defect of a degree sufficiently variant from the average judgment of his fellows in the community he shall be judged irresponsible or incompetent—the phraseology differs with the issues—he shall therefore be declared "insane" and become a warden of the state with respect to his liberty and/or his property.

Let us look for a moment at some of the different

issues, and at a few of the definitions or tests as they are sometimes called. Take the one which gets the front page in the newspapers, namely the responsibility for killing. There are different degrees of killing as we know. Take murder in the first degree. One kills another with knowledge, premeditation and intent. Not in the heat of an angry quarrel, nor by accident nor as an organized member of the police, nor as one of an army of murderers engaged in a war. I am speaking of the purely personal and private kind of murder.

Let us assume that the defense is Insanity. In the first place it is the only defense. Let us say it happened in New York State. Here the statutory definition is short and limited. A man is declared insane in New York State, and therefore declared to be irresponsible and not to be punished by death, if "by reason of mental disease or defect, he does not know the nature and quality of his act and does not know that it is wrong." This seems very clear, but let us assume that he was intoxicated by alcohol or more rarely by thyroid substance, or the delirium of fever, or from too much insulin. There may have been some evidence of premeditation and of hostility yet it does not need much arguing to realize that an intoxicated or hypoglycemic man does not know the nature and quality of his acts nor know at the time of the act that they are wrong. When as with alcoholic intoxication he himself brought about his mental state he is held responsible. With the other situations there are knotty problems. Even the alcoholic phase might have been a symptom of an epileptic state, as many sprees are, and where are we?

Again let us now suppose that our hypothetical murderer had crossed over to New Jersey and killed his victim there. Now the legal set-up is different in New Jersey. In addition to the right and wrong definition and the knowing test there is added an "ability to control an irresistible impulse." It is not difficult to see that a man who commits murder in New Jersey even if he knew the difference between right and wrong and knew the nature and quality of his acts, yet could not control an irresistible impulse is to be declared insane. In New York he would be sane and responsible and be electrocuted; in New Jersey he would be declared insane and sent to a state hospital. I could give example after example of even more peculiar situations, not only for homicidal activities, but in the making of wills, in the preparation of contracts, and so on, and so on.

I shall not mention names. But once there was a very dramatic murder and a much bruited trial. The defense was that the prisoner was not responsible because of mental disease and should therefore be declared insane. "He did not know the nature and quality of his act nor know that it was wrong at the time of its being committed." The District Attorney claimed that he did know the nature and quality of his act and did know that it was wrong and he therefore should be declared to be sane, responsible and punishable. In the middle of the trial the same District Attorney demanded that a Committee be appointed to judge if the prisoner was competent to be tried. Whether or not, on this new issue, he was or was not to be declared "insane." Now the test in this new issue, in brief, is that a man must be an idiot or an imbecile or in such a state of confusion as not to know anything in order that he should not be able to confer with his counsel in the preparation of his defense. Here was a pretty pickle. A prosecuting officer who on the one hand was declaring that a prisoner was of a superlative degree of intelligence—for who of us knows the difference between right and wrong—and yet at the same time, and in the same court-room, and in the same hour, was declaring the prisoner was such an idiot or imbecile as not to be able to confer with his counsel in the preparation of his defense. The law in its relation to matters of psychiatry is full of such dumb-cluck tricks, and to pull their own chestnuts out of the fire the lawyers roar about the venial experts, the alienists. Here may it be interpolated that the word alienist is also a legal word and refers to expert psychiatric opinion in a court. To speak of a psychiatrist as an alienist outside of this special type of activity is nonsense.

The particular hot chestnut that the lawyer is anxious to have the alienist pull out of the fire for him and get burned is in the matter of the procedure on evidence. Such procedure permits the counsel of one side to paint one picture of the situation, just as one looks at one side of a coin, and then permits the opposing counsel to turn the coin over and picture the opposite side. This is a trifle out of focus but in essence this is the chief reason why the public are fed with the picture of conflicts among experts. The public does not know the legal tricks and are always hoodwinked. The hypothetical question is one of these monstrous legal tricks. It describes some one who never existed, never could exist, and is usually a farce from beginning to end.

This is but one of the innumerable absurdities in legal procedure which have existed for centuries and which undoubtedly had something to do with the judgment of Dickens, in his time, that the "law was an ass." I shall not set myself up as knowing more than Charles Dickens.

I shall go no further in the discussion of this highly important background, the intrusion of anachronistic legal conceptions for the solving of medical problems. I would but insist that as a very material part of the social fabric, which is as riddled with pock-marks of incompetency as were the citizens of London with smallpox in Shakespeare's day, it is of supreme importance to remember that such aspects of the environment play a large part in the conflicts that are going on in the human psyche and that grave departures from the ideal of the law, namely Justice, are among the most potent factors in the causation of psychiatric problems.

However, here and there one finds indications of better things. In the days of William Shakespeare even Queen Elizabeth was pock-marked along with the majority of her subjects. It is a far cry to hope that a control of the poxes of Injustice comparable to that of smallpox may come in the next three hundred years as has happened in the past same span of time for this infectious disease.

Now let us consider something less nebulous than the millennium of Universal Justice, a subject dear to the poet, the philosopher, the theologian and the office-seeking politician. Let us take a peep at Bedlam [4] itself, as I promised to earlier. If I have made my meaning clear, psychiatry, however, deals with a far wider range of behavior reaction than those biological distortions—which the tool of classification at present calls psychoses—under the terms schizophrenia, epilepsy, manic-depressive, general paralysis, compulsion neurosis, hysteria, and so on, and for which present-day social economic necessities have devised schemes for housing and for treating. To the popular mind psychiatry is that branch of medicine that deals with the study and treatment of gross mental disease, and to that same popular mind, as in the days of Shakespeare, to take a peep at Bedlam for a penny or tuppence, or whatever the charge happened to be, embodied a view of the bizarre behavior of the lunatic. Readers may recall that John Evelyn in his *Diary* writes of finding the lunatics in chains (1657). This was in the old Bishopsgate Hospital, some ten years before the new hospital designed by Robert Hooke was erected in Moorfields. Liverpool Street Railroad Station now occupies the ancient site of Bedlam. Pepys, a Governor of the

[4] *See* E. G. O'Donoghue, *The Story of Bethlehem Hospital from its Foundation in 1247* (New York, 1915).

Hospital (1662) in his equally interesting record has much of interest to say about Bedlam. It was a regular show in those days, every day save Sunday was visiting day, and as mentioned there was a fee. True it might be only a penny but one year it brought in an income of about £400 which meant, at a penny a time, nearly a hundred thousand visitors. At one time Shakespeare lived right around the corner and I have little doubt that he spent much time there. So also did Thomas Dekker, who, the reader will remember, staged one of his plays as of Bedlam.

Richard Burton of Christ's College, Oxford, was the author of *The Anatomy of Melancholy* which was published at about the same time. It is a classic in that all of the opinions of all the ancients regarding mental diseases can be found therein, but it cannot be compared with Shakespeare for actual case material. Burton was a bookworm and never saw Bedlam; Shakespeare and Dekker were actual observers.

Severe mental diseases such as we find to-day undoubtedly existed among the folk even of the old stone age. Many lower animals in fact behave at times in ways comparable to psychotic behavior in man. Thus the comparative psychologist speaks in the Homeric strain. I have no doubt that the large group of psychoses, which, following the classification of the American Psychiatric Association are known as the toxic, infectious, and exhaustion psychoses were comparatively frequent in prehistoric times, since famine was ever imminent, war incessant, and the conflict with the elements furious and unabating.

I have intimated that I shall not detail any history of psychiatry in the narrow sense of the description of the symptoms, and the modes of treatment of the mentally ill. I shall skip all allusions to Hippocrates, Empedocles, Aristotle, Plato, Galen, Celsus, and Aretæus. All of these may be found fully detailed in Burton. Moreover I shall not narrate the innumerable weird and eccentric ideas about mental disorders that have been held through the ages, from the primitive demons and devils, the gnomes and elves and witches; nor any of the superstitious riff-raff that clutters the pages of history. Even the men of the old stone age had the idea that there was something in the head, for they trephined the skull to let out whatever it was they thought was bothering the individual. The masked demons of the past with their dances and the priestly exorcisms and incantations, these are ancient history and well known. If even a king, like Nebuchadnezzar, was turned out to grass as a mode of therapy or neglect I suspect that then, even as to-day, there were wandering hordes of psychotic hoboes, "lunatic lollers," is what they are termed in *Piers Plowman* (whose author himself roamed with the Toms of Bedlam (1337)).

Nor shall I bore you with the description of the temples of Æsculapius, nor of the numerous healing resorts to which the ill in spirit flocked then as to-day. One shining bit comes to us in the life of the poet Horace that may be worth noting. Horace was probably a manic-depressive type. In his depressions he went to the island of Anticyra and we have a fragment of his lament lest he should get well and have to leave this delightful spot. Hearsay has it that Anticyra was a spot where the plant *Hyoscyamus* was indigenous. It has been one of the favorite remedies for mental disturbance, especially of the restless and noisy, since the days of Hippocrates and to-day, as hyoscine, is widely used for quieting noisy patients. It induces pleasant visions as do opium and alcohol, still old reliable remedies as in the days of long ago.

I have already intimated that the Greeks of the days of Pericles had analyzed the mental disorders into many fine subtle categories. Many of their names are still used but it must not be forgotten that these ancient names do not correspond in meaning with the same terms that are in use to-day.

In one important aspect the Greeks were very modern. They had a highly intuitive sense about the causation of certain mental disorders especially of the significance of heredity. This heredity of the Greeks was good genetics. It was founded on the evils of consanguineous matings. Out of the unconscious storehouse of experience there arose a definite attitude towards incestuous unions. We know that even more primitive peoples had highly complicated incest taboos. Frazer has given us a four-volume work on exogamy and endogamy relative to such unconscious attitudes. But the Greek dramatists, for the first time, dragged the evil into the open light of conscious thought. It then became an attribute of the Ego of the race and has operated as a defense mechanism ever since. The old term *paranoia,* which still exists in psychiatric parlance, then meant "a mind beside itself" and was caused, as in the case of Œdipus, by what Freud, 2500 years later than Sophocles, called the Œdipus Complex. This means that an unconquered remnant of the incestuous and parricidal impulses with which mankind universally had to struggle, had to be modified, either by sublimation or by some biological distortion expressed through some disease process. I might even call attention to a bit of prehistory relative to incest in plant life. Evidently many of the plants had learned the advantages of cross-fertilization.

I can touch but very briefly upon the gradual development of the institutional care of the mentally ill from the turning out to grass method to the growth of such institutions as the New York Psychiatric Institute, the Payne Whitney Clinic, Bloomingdale, Hartford Retreat, the Phipp's Clinic or St. Elizabeths of Washington, D. C., and other similar hospitals now universally distributed. They are all comparatively modern. So far as my reading goes the Arabs, in Persia, were the first to build mental hospitals in the modern sense of the word. As early as the fifth to sixth centuries there was a flourishing school at Jundishapur where Greek medicine was taught. It flourished five to six centuries and had special psychiatric wards or buildings. In medieval days the psychotics wandered, were confined in fool cages, or shut up in garrets or cellars. Many were in the almshouses, prisons, or with the leprous and the criminals.

In a recent very charming drama, under the title

Princess Isabelle, Maeterlinck has given a delightful picture of the city of Gheel in Belgium where, from perhaps as early as the ninth century, mentally ill people have been taken into individual homes and cared for as members of the family. Gheel so functions to-day, and Maeterlinck's picture is not overdrawn. Bedlam, discussed earlier, was begun in the middle of the twelfth century first as a religious hospice for the Brothers of St. Mary of Bethlehem. Other institutions slowly began to be erected in Europe. It will not be possible here to detail these matters further, notwithstanding much interesting historical material. I mention them only as a part of the picture which, because of their fixed and not unformidable structure outside and even more inside, has built up a widespread attitude of dread and fear quite unwarranted in reality.

I fear that I have given but a very meager and fragmentary sketch of the historical and prehistorical backgrounds of psychiatry. I have left out so much about magic and superstition, about the infinitely varying series of theories concerning the origins and therapy of mental disorders, about sorcery and the demons and the devils, the spirits, the gnomes, and the witches, and the lurid history of the grotesque ideas of possession, demoniacal and otherwise. I have intentionally called attention to quite a different group of thoughts. These have clustered about the conception of the all-important pervading influence of the psyche in the biological function of adaptation of the human animal to reality, that is, the forces of his external environment and to the inner drives of his organic needs and satisfactions. I have tried to emphasize not only the ancient maxim, *Mens sana in corpore sano*—a healthy mind in a healthy body—but also, and here with increasing accent, the additional maxim—I shall not latinize it—"a healthy body in a healthy mind."

Here again an ancient Greek has shown the way. Democritus,[5] the father of the atomic theory, wrote, "It is meet for men to take account of the soul rather than the body, for perfection of soul corrects wretchedness of the bodily tabernacle, but bodily strength without reasoning makes the soul not a whit better."

[5] Democritus. Diehl, *Fragmenta.* 187, p. 419. *See* Scroon, p. 221.

II

THE MECHANISMS OF HEREDITY

BY

CHARLES R. STOCKARD, M.D.

PROFESSOR OF ANATOMY, CORNELL UNIVERSITY MEDICAL COLLEGE

II

THE MECHANISMS OF HEREDITY

THIS subject is of interest since our presence in the world is without doubt a result of such mechanisms. We have been derived from a continuous stream of life which probably reaches completely back to the beginning of life on this earth. The truth of this statement depends upon the certainty that each generation of living beings arises as offspring from a previous generation. No one now imagines an organism as arising spontaneously rather than from existing living stuff, though such a view was frequently held in earlier days.

Generations are constantly arising and dying away, but the germ plasm from which they originate forms a continuous stream of life. The idea of the continuity of the germ plasm was forcibly presented by the German zoölogist, August Weismann, during the latter decades of the last century.

The central fact in such a concept is that we do not truly inherit from the bodies or soma of our parents, nor do we transmit the individual characters of our own bodies to our children. Children resemble their parents on account of the fact that they arise from a combination of the same particular lines of germ plasm which had given rise to the parents themselves. The individual serves as host or nurse for the germinal material which was handed down from the previous generation, and his characters as such produce little if any effect upon the germ. We realize further that this germinal material can only develop under limited environmental conditions. For example, simply raising or lowering the temperature to certain degrees will quickly destroy it.

Many such facts were appreciated in a general way at the end of the last century, but all our more accurate and detailed knowledge of heredity has come since 1900. The serious study of heredity by experimental methods began with this century. DeVries described the mutations of the evening primrose, and Mendel's long-lost laws of heredity were brought to light in 1900. These laws of segregation and redistribution of characters in inheritance gave an accurate basis for experimental analysis. Three years later Sutton, a young student of zoölogy at Columbia, pointed out with striking detail and correctness the probable associations between the sorting and redistribution of characters following Mendel's two laws of heredity and the behavior and distribution of small bodies called chromosomes in the maturation stages of the egg and sperm cells. These brilliant discoveries of the behavior of characters in inheritance and the associated behavior of the chromosomes in the germ cells initiated the remarkable series of parallel investigations in genetics and cytology which have so rapidly built up our present understanding of the mechanisms of heredity.

THE INHERITANCE AND EXPRESSION OF CHARACTERS

To illustrate the inheritance and development of characters we may consider as a concrete case the wide variation in number of digits or toes found in different animals. The feet of the primitive ancestral land-living vertebrate animals had five digits. In evolution the vertebrate foot has become specialized in various ways and has tended to reduce the number of toes. The loss of toes reaches extreme limits in the hoofed mammals until the horse possesses only one well developed digit, and walks on its third toe-nail. In the guinea-pig there are four toes on the front foot and only thee on the hind foot; the thumb has disappeared in front and the little toe and great toe behind. In many races of guinea-pigs an extra toe frequently appears on the hind foot in the position of the original little toe or fifth digit. When such a stock of guinea-pigs is carefully selected and bred a well developed little toe may be regained on the hind foot, and in these animals the thumb at times reappears on the front foot, thus bringing back the old complete five-fingered condition of the front foot. The reappearance of the toes which had fallen out in evolution shows that there is still present in the germ the original basis for their inheritance.

In dogs there are five toes on the front foot and usually only four toes on the hind foot; the great toe is missing, just the condition finally brought back in the guinea-pig. In many dog breeds the great toe reappears on the hind foot as the so-called dew claw. When this toe reappears it is interesting to find that it is often doubled; thus the hind foot, which usually has only four toes, instead of regaining a single toe and returning to the original five, actually becomes six-toed. The great toe in the dog is in the process of being lost, and the doubling is an indication of this degenerate tendency.

Extra digits in human families have been followed through several generations and in some of these families with supernumerary digits there has been found a tendency among other members to reduce the number of digits. The occurrence of extra or supernumerary digits seems to be the early indication of a tendency to reduce the digit number as has so frequently occurred among mammals. The reappearance of digits which have been absent for numbers of generations clearly indicates that the hereditary background for the absent digits is still present in the germ plasm and the failure to express these digits is probably due to some shift in balance among the hereditary factors having to do with the determination of the fingers and toes.

There are many common examples to illustrate the fact that although a particular character is definitely inherited, it may not be developed or expressed in the body of the individual, and thus from general observation its presence would not be suspected. To illustrate, the male of the Sebright bantam fowl is normally always hen-feathered. The feathers on the neck are short and not gaily colored hackles; the tail and saddle feathers are straight and short. The comb and wattles of this male are large and fully developed as in the ordinary cock. If the Sebright male be caponized he promptly develops a new plumage, exhibiting the gay colors and long sickle feathers of the rooster, but at the same time the handsome comb and wattles become reduced and the head furnishings now resemble those of the hen. It is thus evident that this male fowl inherits cock plumage, but in his usual body environment the rooster style plumage is suppressed and only hen-feathering is developed. The characters of an animal are not only dependent upon the qualities inherited, but also upon the conditions under which these qualities develop.

Modifying the composition of sea-water in which the eggs of fishes develop will cause the development of the eggs to be changed in various ways. The characters of an individual developing from an egg may be modified also by an unusual temperature change. Flies developed at one temperature may have the normal number of legs whereas the same eggs developing at another temperature will produce flies with supernumerary, or extra, legs. So—as Jennings has expressed it—an animal really does not inherit its characters at all; it simply inherits germinal material from its parents and the characters expressed depend upon the environment in which this germinal material is developed.

These facts suggest a further question as to whether the germ plasm itself may be readily changed by strange environments? One of the early experiments aimed to answer this question was made by Castle on guinea-pigs. The ovaries from an immature black guinea-pig were transplanted into the body of a young white albino female after her own ovaries had been removed. If normal albino guinea-pigs are mated together, all of their young will be albinos. However, when an albino male was mated to the albino female carrying the ovaries from the black female, three offspring were produced, and all of them were black. Thus the hereditary basis for pigmentation in the "black ovaries" had not been affected by their sojourn in the white albino female. Many other experiments show the germ plasm to be quite resistant to modification through environmental changes; we shall later consider, however, some treatments which do modify the hereditary material.

NATURE'S CHROMOSOME DEAL AND INHERITED CHARACTERS

It is logical to suppose that the mechanism for inheritance is contained within the cell since all higher plants and animals arise from two united cells, the fertilized seed or egg. What is there in the cell that behaves in such a way as to fit in with the peculiar shifting and sorting of characters which takes place in inheritance? A mechanism comes to light during the divisions of the cell which fits very exactly the demands of the situation, as Sutton originally pointed out. During the ordinary divisions which the cells undergo in growth and development small dark-staining bodies appear in the nucleus in definite numbers.

Every one of these dark structures divides longitudinally into two equal parts and the two halves separate and pass one into each of the two daughter cells. Thus the number of these nuclear bodies, called chromosomes, is constantly maintained in every cell of the individual.

In the germ cells there is, in addition to the ordinary method of splitting the chromosomes and retaining their full number, a peculiar maturation division. At this maturation division the chromosomes show themselves to exist in pairs of similar kinds. One member of each pair was derived from the maternal parent and the other member from the paternal. These similar chromosomes, one from each parent, fuse together so that the entire number of chromosomes is apparently reduced to half; each chromosome, however, is double. The two members of each pair later separate from one another, one entire member going to one cell and the other to the sister cell. In this way, each cell receives only half of the original number of single chromosomes. The mature germ cell containing half the chromosome number is then fertilized by uniting with a cell from the opposite sex also containing half the number. Through fertilization of the egg the original number of chromosomes is restored and a new individual begins its development. For example, when a cell contains six chromosomes we recognize these as being three pairs; one member of each pair has been derived from the mother and one member from the father. When the germ cells of this individual mature to form eggs, the maternal and paternal chromosomes pair and subsequently separate to be redistributed in many different combinations among these eggs; that is, all of the maternal chromosomes are not likely to pass into one cell nor all of the paternal into the other, but the chance is that all possible mixtures of maternal and paternal chromosomes will occur among a large number of eggs. The same is true, of course, for the male sperm cells. A careful study of Figure I, will make the process clear.

Pairing of the chromosomes, called synapsis, and subsequent separation of the members of the pairs in the maturation of the germ cells, is one of the most important phenomena in biology. Montgomery long ago pointed out that this chromosomal pairing may be thought of as the last step completing in detail the union of the egg and sperm and this only takes place when the individual is mature and now preparing to produce the next generation. There is much evidence to indicate that deep-lying influences are exerted by one chromosome upon the other during this pairing.

The sorting and shifting of the chromosomes may be understood more clearly by considering a concrete case. For example, suppose a species carries in its cells four chromosomes, a pair of rod-shaped and a pair of dot-like ones. A female of this species pure for two characters determined by these chromosomes may be mated with a male that is pure for two contrasted characters. We may show the chromosomes of the female in light color and those of the male in dark, see again Figure I. When the eggs of the female are mature and ready to be fertilized they will each contain one light bar chromosome and one light dot, while the mature sperm of the male each contain one dark bar and one dark dot. On fertilization, the eggs and sperm cells unite giving rise to the new generation, each cell of which will contain four chromosomes, a pair of rods, one light and one dark, and a pair of dots, one light and one dark. Thus, every individual of the F_1 generation has exactly the same chromosomal composition, and differs in its composition from each of the two parents. The F_1s are all similar in appearance and resemble in their several characters the parent with the dominant characters. When these similar, F_1, animals become mature, they will form not similar but four different kinds of eggs in equal numbers, and four different kinds of sperm in equal numbers on the basis of chromosomal compositions, see third line from bottom in Figure I. One fourth of the number of eggs will have a gray rod and black dot, another fourth a black rod and gray dot, another a gray rod and dot, and the final fourth a black rod and dot. These are all the combinations possible. The sperm will possess exactly the same four kinds of chromosomal combinations. We may assume that each kind of egg is likely to be fertilized by any one of the four kinds of sperm thus giving rise to a second filial generation of the sixteen possible combinations seen in the two bottom lines of Figure I. Four of the sixteen will have the same composition as the F_1 generation, while only one of

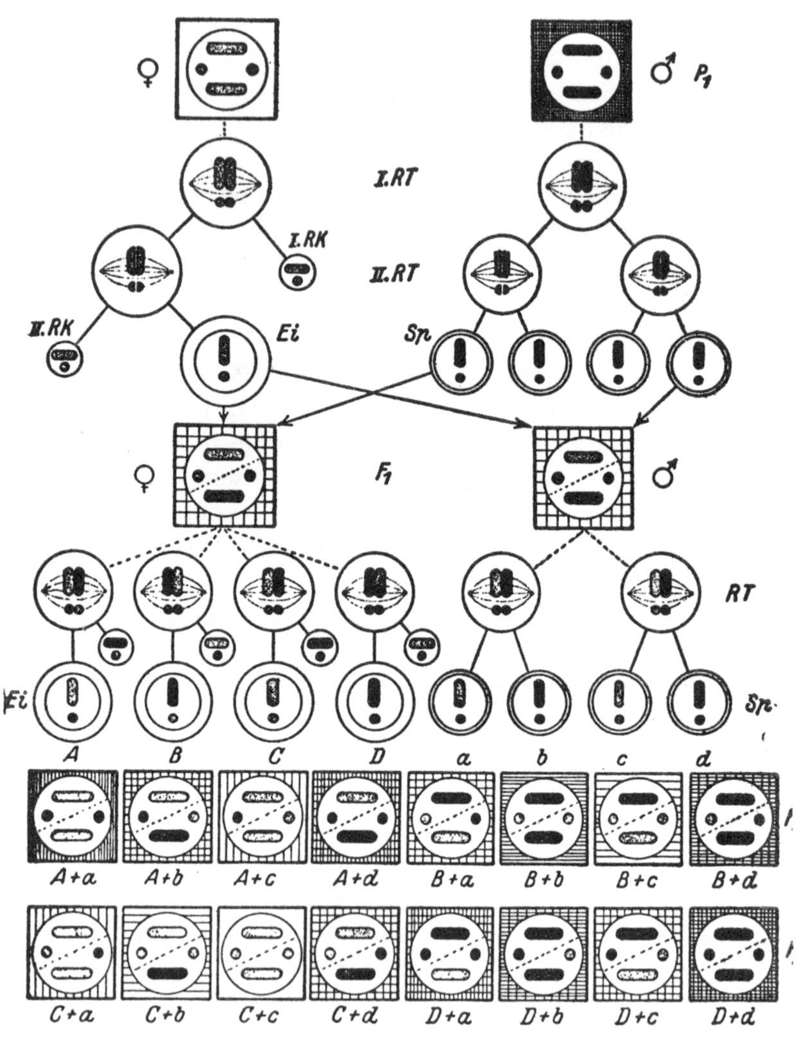

♀
♂
P_1
I. RT
I. RK
II. RT
II. RK
Ei
Sp
♀
F_1
♂
RT
Ei
Sp
A
B
C
D
a
b
c
d
A+a
A+b
A+c
A+d
B+a
B+b
B+c
B+d
C+a
C+b
C+c
C+d
D+a
D+b
D+c
D+d

FIGURE 1.—DIAGRAM OF CROSSING TWO ANIMALS, EACH WITH TWO PAIRS OF CHROMOSOMES CARRYING CONTRASTED QUALITIES AS INDICATED BY THE GRAY RODS AND DOTS AND THE BLACK RODS AND DOTS.

The first offspring, F_1, in center of diagram all inherit one gray and one black rod and dot; all inheric exactly the same composition. When mature, they will produce four kinds of eggs or four kinds of sperm as indicated in the fourth and third lines from the bottom. Any one of the four kinds of sperm may fertilize any one of the four kinds of eggs and sixteen different individual combinations will be produced in the F_2 generation as shown in the two bottom rows of squares. Only one of these sixteen, third in lower line, is of the same constitution as the grandmother and one, last in lower line, is the same as the grandfather for the two pairs of chromosomes. Four have the same constitution as the F_1 parents and ten show new combinations of the four chromosomes. *After* K. BELAR.

the sixteen shows the original constitution of the pure female with which we started, and similarly only one of the sixteen has the identical constitution of the original male. All the other ten individuals have compositions differing not only from the original grandparents, but from their immediate F_1 parents as well. In this F_2 generation we have ten out of sixteen individuals with new combinations of the four chromosomes and consequently with new constitutions, but all ten of these are not different from one another. Thus F_2 animals derived from crossing two stocks contrasted in two sets of characters furnish a series of combinations of these characters; many of the combinations are new and peculiar. An F_1 mother and father frequently produce a litter showing great constitutional differences among the individuals in spite of the fact that all members of this litter develop in the same environment and after birth may be subject to as nearly as possible identical experiences.

These facts are strikingly illustrated by crosses between two pure stocks such as the English bulldog, with a highly modified head and short twisted tail, and the basset-hound, with a normal head and long tail but with short and badly modified extremities. The first generation, F_1, hybrids of this cross are, as would be expected, unlike both parent stocks but are closely similar to one another, which is proof of the purity of the two stocks crossed. The heads of these hybrids are short and heavy-type, the tails are straight and long, and the legs are short and twisted. When these F_1s are bred *inter se* they give rise to an F_2 generation which shows various mixtures of the characters contributed by the two original parent stocks. There are long-legged dogs with hound-like heads but carrying very short, twisted screw-tails. There are basset-legged animals with almost perfect bulldog heads and long hound tails. There also occur new type individuals very unlike their immediate ancestors; some are small midget dogs, while others are quite large with St. Bernard type heads differing very decidedly from the two original stocks from which they were derived. Litter mates differ greatly in size; some are very large, others small, short-legged and dwarf-like. In a series of skulls from this cross-breeding there are among F_2s specimens approaching the bulldog type and others closely approaching the normal basset-hound type. Between these extremes we find a long series of gradations, and also small, midget-like skulls as well as large oversized skulls resembling in type and texture more nearly the skull of a St. Bernard dog than either of the original pure parent types. Frequent structural disharmonies appear among such hybrid animals. A dog may have the long muzzle and upper jaw of the hound with a very short, poorly developed lower jaw and complete misfit of the teeth. These disharmonies would act as lethal conditions in nature, since the individuals are almost unable to grasp food and could not compete for it under natural conditions.

THE CHROMOSOME AS AN ENTIRE UNIT IN INHERITANCE

The cellular mechanism by which various character combinations are brought about may now be considered on the basis of the chromosomes as individual bodies. Every species, as a rule, contains a definite number of chromosomes in all its cells although in many cases the number differs in the two sexes of the same species. The cells of the female contain two sex or X-chromosomes and those of the male only one X-chromosome in many species. The double or paired number of chromosomes, called the diploid or somatic number, varies from as few as four in the cells of the parasitic roundworm *Ascaris* to very great numbers in other species. The number of chromosomes is not definitely connected with degree of complexity or the position of a species in the animal kingdom. In the cells of the human body there are forty-eight chromosomes, twenty-four pairs, while in the cells of the fruit-fly, *Drosophila melanogaster,* which has been the material basis for most of our knowledge of chromosomal behavior in inheritance, there are only four pairs, or eight chromosomes.

The chromosomes not only differ greatly in numbers among species, but there is also enormous differences in their sizes. The four chromosomes of the intestinal worm *Ascaris* are very large compared with the chromosomes of man. Those in certain plants, such as the common pea, are very large, whereas in the jimson-weed and the evening primrose they are quite small; they are also small in the fruit-fly, while in the grasshopper they are large and numerous. The number of chromosomes is usually constant for the species, but this is not always true, particularly among plants where multiples of the usual number are often found. Normally the halved or haploid number is doubled by fertilization to give the normal diploid number with all the chromosomes existing in pairs. In unusual cases the halved or haploid number of chromosomes may be tripled, quadrupled, and so on, forming the so-called triploid condition where there are three of each kind of chromosome in the cells, tetraploid with four of each, and polyploid with many. There may also be extra or additional chromosomes added in peculiar ways.

The fact that the number of chromosomes is usually constant for a species and differs from the numbers in other species is one of the fundamental reasons why hybridization or species crossing is so frequently unsuccessful. For example, if a species with six chromosomes should be crossed with another containing fourteen chromosomes, the reduced numbers of chromosomes would be three and seven respectively. The F_1 hybrids would all contain cells with ten chromosomes. If these hybrids were viable, difficulties would arise in the synapsis of the chromosomes when the maturation of their germ cells took place. The three chromosomes from one parent stock would pair with a more or less similar three from the other stock, but four of the seven chromosomes would be left unpaired. These four odd chromosomes would be sorted in various directions in division, and the combining of germ cells necessary to produce the second filial generation would give rise to many if not all incompatible and non-viable combinations. Differences in chromosomal number is a very important means for preventing the amalgamation and confusion of species. In exceptional cases, however, two varieties with different chromosomal numbers may produce a successful hybrid strain. Ljungdahl crossed two races of cultivated poppies, one with fourteen chromosomes, the reduced number being seven, and the other with seventy chromosomes which reduces to thirty-five; the two reduced numbers combine, giving forty-two chromosomes which arrange themselves agreeably into twenty-one pairs and the hybrid strain is stable and perpetuates itself.

Blakeslee of the Carnegie Institution has discovered many important facts concerning the behavior of chromosomes in his experiments with the common jimson-weed. This plant normally has twelve pairs of chromosomes arranged in typical fashion. The reduced number in both the ovules and pollen grains is twelve single chromosomes. In the jimson-weed there is a decided tendency to form multiples of the chromosomal number in various ways. Blakeslee has classified these conditions into balanced arrangements of haploid with twelve, diploid with twenty-four, triploid with thirty-six, and tetraploid with forty-eight chromosomes. In addition to these there are various unbalanced combinations: haploids with twelve plus one additional chromosome; diploids with minus one or plus one, or plus two similar chromosomes, or plus one of one kind and one of another kind. The triploid and tetraploid types also may be either minus one or more, or plus one or more chromosomes of one or more kinds. The fact that there are multiple and extra chromosomes in the cells of these plants is directly associated with resulting deformities and modifications in stems, leaves and seed pods. Blakeslee has shown very clearly that any modification in the chromosomal number produces a modification and disturbance in the size, shape, and general condition of the resulting plant. The forms of the seed capsules differ greatly in association with the differences in chromosomal composition so that entirely new lines may be built up and developed on this basis.

Not only do entire chromosomes become disarranged in these plants, but in other cases a part of one chromosome becomes attached to an entirely different chromosome. Such shifts of chromosomal pieces are commonly called translocations. Blakeslee has studied extensively a so-called B-race of jimsonweed in which the seventeen half of the chromosome seventeen-eighteen has been transferred to the number one end of the one-two chromosome. Thus the constitutions of the seventeen-eighteen and the one-two chromosomes have both been modified. We shall see later that such changes in chromosomes make it difficult for them to later pair in synapsis with the original normal types from which they were broken.

Studies of these plants clearly show that misplacements and peculiar arrangements of the chromosomes give rise to new and strange forms as stated above. However, these are not the usual things that we commonly see in inheritance. The inheritance of characters as we commonly observe the process may not be dependent upon the chromosome as a whole but rather on certain units located within it.

In some species, as mentioned before, the cells of the female contain two X-chromosomes and those of the male only one. The fact that this chromosome is shuffled in such a way as to accompany or determine the sex of the individuals has been of great advantage in studying its influences on the development of other characters in the body. A simple example will illustrate: There are a great number of different eye colors among the races of the common fruit-fly. The wild type red eye is dominant over a pure white eye and this eye color is determined through the X-chromosome. We may for convenience designate the X-chromosomes in this case as red-X and white-X. When a pure red-eyed female carrying two red X-chromosomes is mated with a white-eyed male which carries only one white X-chromosome, the F_1 hybrids are all red-eyed, the males since they receive their one X only from the red-X mother, and the females since they receive one red-X from the mother which dominates the white-X from the father. When two of these are mated they will produce offspring of several kinds: pure red-eyed females having two X's for red, red-eyed females having a red-X and a white-X, and red-eyed males carrying one red-X and white-eyed males with the one white-X. The color of the eyes is inherited in exactly the same manner as the shifting of the X-chromosomes, and all the females of this generation are red-eyed, and half the males are red-eyed and half white-eyed since red-X dominates white-X.

If we now make the reciprocal cross using to start with a red-eyed male instead of a red-eyed female, the result is very different. In mating a red-eyed male with a pure white-eyed female, we realize that since red is dominant to white this white-eyed female must necessarily carry two white X-chromosomes, and the red-eyed male having only one X must carry the dominant red. All the hybrid males produced by this mating will be white-eyed, and all the females red-eyed. This is due to the fact that all males receive their only X-chromosome from the white-eyed mother, and all the females receive one of the X's from the white-eyed mother and the other X from the red-eyed father, and the dominant red-bearing X causes the females to be red-eyed. In the next generation, from these hybrids we find both red-eyed and white-eyed females in equal numbers and red-eyed and white-eyed males in equal numbers. Here again the eye color has definitely followed the sorting and recombination of the X-chromosomes.

All characters are not, of course, located in the X-chromosome and are not linked or associated with sex. For example, among dogs there is the peculiar mutant condition producing short, twisted legs as is well known in the common dachshund. This short leg results from the influence of a single chromosome, but it is not the sex or X-chromosome. When a short-legged dog is crossed with a normal long-legged type, all of the F_1s of both sexes are short-legged, indicating that the shortness is a simple dominant expression. When these short-legged hybrids are bred together they give rise to a second generation with one-fourth of its members having long legs and three-fourths with short legs, but among the short-legged animals some are shorter than others. The shortest have received two chromosomes carrying the short influence, whereas the intermediate-short have inherited one chromosome for short and one for long; they are mixed or heterozygous for short and are of the same composition so far as this one character goes as the F_1 generation. The second generation gives the typical Mendelian ratio of one pure short: two mixed short: and one pure long. The leg skeletons show very clearly that these three types actually exist and this is crucially proven by the results of crossing the apparently mixed shorts and apparently pure shorts back to the long-legged animal.

Such characters as eye color in Drosophila and leg length in the dogs are thought of as single factor characters. This simply means that their expression follows the distribution of a single chromosome. There are other characters more complex in their inheritance depending upon the distribution of two or more chromosomes. The short screw-tail of the bulldog is such a character. When the short-tailed bulldog is mated to a normal long-tailed dog, all of the first generation hybrids have long tails, showing that the short screwtail is a recessive character. When these long-tailed hybrids are bred together the short screw-tail does not reappear in one out of four individuals but in approximately only one out of sixteen. This indicates that the development of the screw-tail is due to the influence of two recessive factors carried by two different chromosomes. One of the factors we may think of as causing shortening of the tail, and the second factor as causing bending. In such a case as this it is possible to have individuals among the F_2 hybrids with pure inheritance for short and also for straight, thus developing a short straight tail. Others may be pure for bending, but not for short, giving a bent long tail; while only those that are pure for short and bent, having both chromosomes for short and both for bending, have the short bent or screw-tail. In such a double factor case we may have, therefore, different combinations of tail length and shape: (1) the normal, straight long tail; (2) long bent tail; (3) short straight tail; (4) short bent tail. But we actually have more than this on account of the fact that when an animal is pure for short, having two chromosomes for short, and mixed for bent, having one for bent and one for straight, there may be a slight bending of the short tail, due to the presence of the one recessive for bending, and other expressions occur accordingly. The fact is that a character is rarely completely recessive or completely dominant over its antagonist.

Many characters such as head shape, body form, and so on, are dependent upon the influences of a number of factors carried by several different chromosomes. It must be kept in mind that the entire body is influenced in a general way by all these factors. Not only are external features which are readily observed inherited in definite ways, but the quality and type of internal organs are equally characteristic of certain constitutions. For example, the sizes of the thyroid glands differ quite markedly among the various varieties or breeds of dogs. Proportionally the largest thyroid glands are in tiny toy dogs and the relatively smallest glands are found in the giant St. Bernards. It has been found that when a breed with large thyroid is crossed with a small thyroid breed, the inheritance is not a simple affair such as is found for leg length. The thyroid size is a character depending upon multiple factors. It is also found on crossing animals with different sizes of thyroids, that the hybrid generations may have thyroid volumes entirely out of proportion with those from either of the parent stocks. The complex determining the proportional amount of thyroid may be disturbed by crossbreeding so as to give new combinations resulting in most exaggerated proportions.

It is well recognized that the internal secretions from such glands as the thyroid exert profound influences over the growth and development of other body structures, and the genetic analysis of various gland-types is of most fundamental importance in arriving at the function and influence of these secretions, not only in development, but in the economy of the adult animal as well. We have been investigating the inheritance of various internal gland modifications during the past ten years. In this study advantage is taken of the remarkable material supplied by the grossly modified dog breeds. We have interpreted these modifications as being of the kinds often associated with disturbed internal secretions in man. Previous studies on inheritance of various characters in the dog have been made, but none of these investigations aimed at the problems now being studied by us, and the persons conducting those studies—Lange in Switzerland, Plate in Germany, Little in this country, and others—have made no reference whatever to the association between the internal secretions and the peculiarly modified structures in the few animals they have used. The inheritance of variations in internal secretions and chemical differences among breeds is a field demanding much investigation and one in which only little has been done.

LETHAL CHARACTERS AND INHERITANCE OF DEATH

Morgan and his school, in genetic studies with the fruit-fly, have found a great number of so-called lethal characters, and others have discovered similar conditions in a number of animals. By lethal is meant a constitutional condition incapable of complete development so that specimens with such inheritance die during early stages of development or before adult life is reached. There are probably many cases of hereditary lethals among higher animals.

We have recently found in breeding certain giant dogs that a most peculiar multiple factor lethal appears. Individuals which carry only a part of the necessary group of factors are not affected. Three different breeds have been found to carry the several factors necessary for the lethal effects. When normally strong St. Bernard dogs have been mated with normal great Danes, the hybrid offspring develop a peculiar paralytic condition at about three months of age. A study of the spinal cord in these paralyzed puppies shows death of anterior-horn motor nerve cells in the lumbar region. This loss of nerve cells causes the paralysis of certain muscle groups in the hind legs. Breeding experiments indicate the condition to be caused by the combination of at least three dominant hereditary factors. When only one or two of the factors are present, the animal is unaffected, but when all three factors occur in either mixed or pure combinations the animal becomes paralyzed. The degree of paralysis varies, depending upon whether the three dominant factors concerned are present in pure, double or mixed combinations.

We have, in this case, an hereditary length of life of only three months for certain motor nerve cells in the spinal cord in contrast to the fact that the other cells in such an animal may continue to live and function for the usual dog's life-span of ten to twelve years. The possibility is suggested that the length of life in many animal species may be determined by a definitely inherited life-span for some one vital organ or tissue while other body tissues in such an animal might be constituted to live for many years beyond this time. For example, should a species inherit a life-span of only five years for its kidney cells, the death of this vital organ would necessarily determine the end of life for the entire body. It is well known that the length of life is quite definite for most species. A mouse is old at two years, a rat at three, a dog at ten or twelve, a horse at twenty, and the human being at seventy. The constitution of each species seems to be definitely limited in its life-span, and a more complete knowledge of hereditary lethals may aid in understanding the limiting cause.

UNITS WITHIN THE CHROMOSOMES

Thus far we have associated the inheritance of characters with the distribution of the chromosomes as total bodies. It has long been known that certain groups of characters are almost constantly associated or linked together in inheritance and it has been assumed that each chromosome influences the expression of these associated or linked character groups. It was later discovered that from time to time some of the characters of a linked group might become freed and appear independent of the original group. The fact that characters are linked and that occasionally this linkage is broken gives reason to believe that chromosomes may also break, and further that smaller units contained within the chromosomes are the elements which influence the development of the characters. These elements in the chromosomes are called genes. The study of the behavior of the genes in inheritance is the field of genetics.

The genic composition of an individual plant or animal is termed its genotype, and the bodily characteristics of the individual make up its phenotype. The phenotype may not completely supply evidence of the entire genotype. The genotype may contain many recessive elements which are only discovered through breeding. Also, identical genotypes do not give rise to the same phenotype in all environments.

Every chromosome is thought to be a series of genes arranged in linear fashion comparable to beads on a string. The chromosomes exist in pairs and when the members of a pair come together during synapsis, the string of genes in one chromosome is thought to aline exactly with the genes of its mate. The pairing of chromosomes during synapsis is actually a pairing of the genes. The two genes of a pair are called allelomorphs. When these two genes are similar, the cell is pure or homozygous for their effects. For example, if each of the genes influencing the production of blue eye color are present, then the individual has a constitution pure or homozygous for blue eyes. If the two allelomorphic genes of the pair are dissimilar, then the individual is mixed or heterozygous for their effects and the expression of the character which these genes affect will be more largely influenced by one of the genes than by the other. The one gene is dominant, the other recessive in competition with one another. Continuing the example, if one gene of the eye-color pair is the determiner for black eyes and the other gene of the pair determines blue eye color, an individual carrying these genes is mixed in its genotype for eye color, but will develop black eyes since the black gene dominates the blue. Breeding such a mixed black-eyed individual with a blue-eyed mate will disclose the recessive blue gene in the mixed parent since half of the offspring will inherit a gene for blue from each parent and will be blue eyed whereas a pure black-eyed parent will have only black-eyed children by a blue-eyed mate.

A single gene not only affects or influences a single character in the body of the individual, but each gene very probably exerts an influence over all the characters of the individual. A given gene, however, does tend to produce more effect on a certain character than do other genes. The gene for blue eyes has a special effect on the pigmentation of the eye, but it also has certain general effects on other parts of the body though these are not so readily detected. Again, the effect a gene produces in a given combination may not be quite the same as the effect it produces in another. A change of the position of a gene in the general gene series changes its association with other genes and probably modifies its action.

CROSSING-OVER OR GENE-SWAPPING BETWEEN CHROMOSOMES

Chromosomes in many cases bend and twist around one another during the pairing or synapsis. While in such positions a piece of one chromosome may be

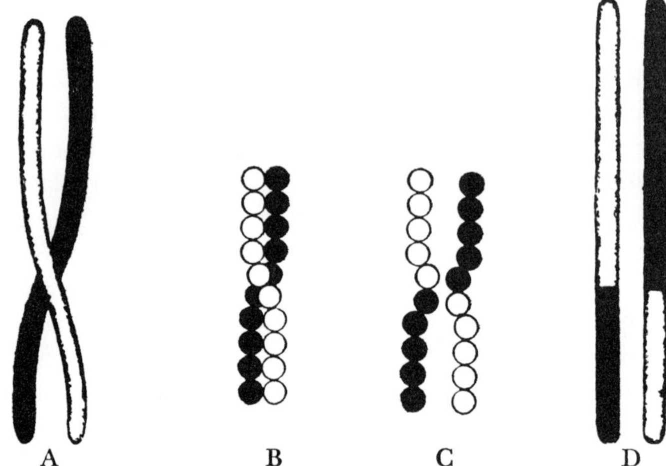

FIGURE 2.—DIAGRAM OF CROSSING-OVER, OR THE EXCHANGE OF PARTS, BETWEEN TWO CHROMOSOMES.

A and D illustrate the result on the entire chromosome. B and C illustrate the regrouping of the individual genes in crossing-over. *After* T. H. MORGAN.

exchanged for a corresponding portion of the other. Such happenings are termed crossing-over. A group of genes from each chromosome crosses over into the other, or swaps places, see Figure 2. If these genes are dissimilar in the two chromosomes, then it is readily seen that new linkage groups of characters will be established by each of the newly constituted chromosomes. This breaking of the series of genes in the chromosomes has been a most fortunate phenomenon in enabling students of genetics to accurately locate the position of a definite gene. The frequency of gene crossing-over has been calculated in hundreds of cases. To illustrate a case of crossing-over, if a normal gray, long-winged fruit-fly be mated with a peculiar black-bodied rudimentary-winged fly, the hybrid offspring will all be normal gray, long-winged flies since normal gray and long wings dominate black color and rudimentary wings, shown in Figure 3. When such a gray, long-winged hybrid female is mated with the rudimentary-winged black male like its father, we should then obtain offspring in equal numbers normal gray and rudimentary black. Instead of this we get the surprising result of only 82 per cent of the offspring showing this distribution, while the remaining 18 per cent are divided into two equal classes of new type gray individuals with rudimentary wings and new type long-winged but black individuals, shown at bottom of Figure 3. This occurrence results from the fact that during the synapsis of the chromosomes in the hybrid female, crossing-over between the genes for black and gray as well as between genes for long-winged and rudimentary-winged takes place in 18 per cent of the pairing chromosomes. The usual linkage of the characters is broken apart and the new combinations occur.

The greater the distance apart two genes lie in the chromosome, the more likely they are to become separated from one another by crossing-over, and conversely, the closer together two genes lie, the more unlikely they are to be broken apart as a result of crossing-over. On the basis of the relation between distance apart and the probability of becoming sep-

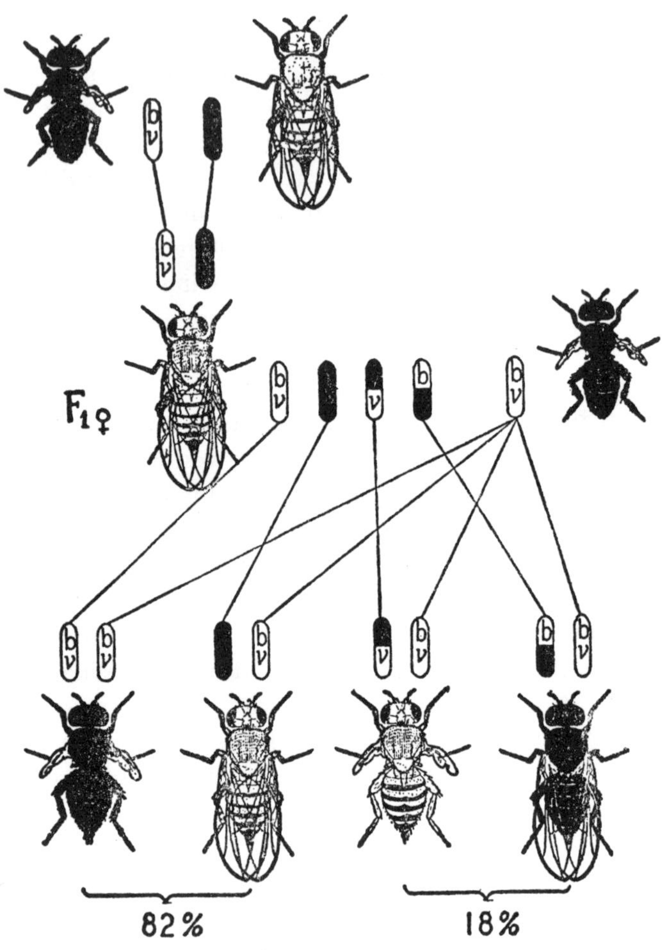

FIGURE 3.—CROSS BETWEEN BLACK VESTIGIAL AND GRAY LONG-WINGED, WILD-TYPE FLY.

Crossing-over occurs in the F_1 ♀. Eighty-two per cent of her eggs contain chromosomes similar to those received from her parents but in 18 per cent there has occurred crossing-over of the b and v as the diagram shows. *After* T. H. MORGAN.

arated by crossing-over, the exact position of a large number of genes has been located in the chromosomes. The maps of gene positions in the four chromosomes of the fruit-fly *Drosophila melanogaster* have been plotted in very complete detail and with experimentally demonstrated accuracy.

NATURE OF THE GENE

From the above considerations we are led to the view that the mechanism of inheritance largely resolves itself into the arrangements of the qualitatively different genes in the chromosomes of the cell nucleus. Important questions arise: What is a gene? How do genes maintain themselves in the definite linear arrangement in the chromosome? Up to the present time an individual gene has not been handled or analyzed. One may presume, however, that it is a complex organic molecule or a group of such molecules. The large-chain and side-chain molecules which organic chemistry richly supplies fill quite completely the pattern we might imagine for the gene. Such a molecule, for example, may react somewhat differently in different environments or in different mixtures. In a similar way, a gene may not bring about the same effects in different environments. If, for example, we consider the gene most concerned in producing the short leg in the dogs discussed before, we find that when this gene is carried into the cells of breeds having different proportions and textures of bone the degree of influence of the gene on the bone pattern and leg length is not always the same. The long slender bone of the greyhound is not so strongly modified as is the less slender bone of the shepherd-dog or the coarser textured bone of the bulldog. The function of a gene is influenced by the genic complex in which it exists.

Genes must necessarily possess a certain degree of stability and yet if characters are continually changing in evolution with new things occurring there must also necessarily be some possibility for change or modifications in the genes themselves. If the gene is a complex organic molecule it is then possible to understand how it may become changed in spite of its tendency to remain stable. It is well known that many large organic molecules with a chain or side-chain pattern may be caused to split off secondary molecules and the loss of these necessarily modifies the character of the original molecule. We may hold hypothetically that the so-called mutations in gene composition occur in a similar manner.

Gene mutations are known to take place in somatic or body cells as well as in the germ cells of both plants and animals. In the common garden delphinium there is a lavender strain which occasionally shows blossoms spotted with purple. These purple spots are due to the fact that the dominant lavender gene in some way has become changed so as to allow the recessive purple influence to express itself. There is also a rose strain of delphinium in which the same thing occurs, giving very fine purple specking. The mutation in the lavender strain occurs during an earlier period in the development of the blossom and this gives the larger purple spots on account of the fact that more cells are derived from the cell in which the mutation occurred. If the mutation occurs at a later stage in the development of the blossom there are only a few cell generations afterwards produced and the purple area resulting is only a small speck instead of a large spot. Somatic mutations occur in pigmented regions of certain animals and here again the recessive color appears as a spot. Such mutations as these are only transmitted to the daughter cells in this area of the body and since the mutation may not occur in the germ cells, no effect on the offspring from this spotted individual will be observed.

Mutations also occur in the germ cell of the reproductive glands and these bring about modifications in the following generations. In this way entirely new characters arise in the race. The egg changes before the hen. Several hundred germinal mutations have been discovered in the common fruit-fly. There are eleven different mutations which modify the wings, either as to size, shape, or position, and these new characters are inherited in typical Mendelian ratios when the modified flies are crossed with the usual wild-type individual.

Mutations are frequently occurring in nature since they are found in all plants and animals that have been carefully studied for such occurrences. Mutations have been artificially brought about by subjecting the germ cells of animals to X-ray and other radiations. As a result of such treatment the rate of mutation is enormously increased. All effects of X-ray treatments are not confined to individual genes but breaks in the chromosomes and dislocations of large pieces of the chromosomes frequently result. A part of one chromosome may be translocated and become attached to another chromosome of a different pair; in this way one chromosome loses a piece containing a certain number of its genes and these become added to the other chromosome. When breeding an animal carrying such chromosomes with a normal mate it is evident that some of the offspring will be deficient in a certain series of genes while an equal number of the offspring will possess an additional group of genes. Such disbalance in the genic constitutions always brings about modifications in the development and expression of the characteristics of the resulting animal if it be able to develop at all.

Treatment with X-ray may also knock out or destroy middle portions of the chromosome, producing so-called deleted conditions. A certain number of the genes at the two ends of the chromosome remain and those occupying the middle region are missing. The effects of this are also readily analyzed by breeding such treated individuals to normal mates. By means of these experiments the accuracy of the chromosome maps which were originally drawn from studies on character linkage and crossing-over have been confirmed in considerable detail.

GENES IN GIANT CHROMOSOMES

Our knowledge of the nature and position of the genes in the chromosomes has recently been greatly increased by an entirely new method of attack. For unknown reasons the chromosomes in the cells of the salivary glands in a number of insects become enormously enlarged both in width and in length. They are truly giant chromosomes. The recent studies of these chromosomes were initiated by Painter at the University of Texas. These enormous chromosomes with their peculiarly banded appearance were first discovered long ago. Balbiani in 1881 and Leidig in 1883 observed giant chromosomes in the larva of the chironomus fly. Van Herwerden in 1910 again observed them in the same animal. Erhard in 1911 and Alverdes in 1912 studied them. However, all these earlier observers were completely unable to appreciate the meaning of the dots and bands on the chromosomes as is now possible in the light of our knowledge of the chromosome map.

In the hands of Painter the banding on these giant chromosomes suggests an entirely new significance: the bands are closely related to the genes. After careful study Painter was able to identify the different regions of these giant salivary-chromosomes as comparable with known regions of the tiny germ-cell chromosomes in Drosophila. He then made another remarkable and extremely fortunate discovery: the giant chromosomes in the cells of the salivary glands pair in a synapsis exactly as occurs in the reduction division of the germ cells. This pairing turns out to be highly useful since it makes possible a comparison of the arrangements and positions of the genes in the two chromosomes of the pair. All discrepancies in gene position occurring in the two chromosomes may be detected.

Painter crossed *Drosophila melanogaster* with *D. simulans* and discovered that the genes were not identically arranged in the comparable chromosomes of the two species, and on this account the two chromosomes of a pair were unable to go into synapsis at certain places throughout their length. Painter also crossed normal flies with mates that had been treated with X-rays so as to produce translocations and deletions of certain parts of their chromosomes. The hybrids resulting showed striking pictures in the synapsis of their salivary-gland chromosomes. A deleted chromosome would pair with the normal chromosome in synapsis so as to place their comparable allelomorphic genes exactly opposite and when a place was reached which corresponded to the deleted part of the treated chromosome the normal chromosome was thrown into a loop since there were no comparable genes in the treated chromosome with which the genes of this portion were able to pair. By crossing such flies it was possible to identify the group of genes which had been deleted from the treated chromosome.

The study of individual genes in the giant chromosomes has been further advanced by the striking experiments of Dobzshanski on crosses between *Droso-*

phila pseudobscura and *D. miranda.* These two species or varieties are so nearly alike that it is very difficult to distinguish between them. Yet in the giant chromosomes of the hybrids Dobzshanski found that the gene arrangements in the two members of the pairs differed greatly in a variety of ways as was plainly shown during synapsis. Certain genes which are located in a given chromosome in one of these species are actually found located in a different chromosome in the other. The sequence of the genes in certain cases was reversed in the chromosome of one species as compared with their positions in the other.

As mentioned before, the influence or function of a gene is probably modified through changes in its relative position. For example, if genes are arranged in a series *a, b, c, d, e, f,* the *a* gene may function quite differently when this series is broken and reversed so as to place the *a* next to *f,* as *e, d, c, b, a, f*—this has been found experimentally. Modifications of gene arrangement in comparable chromosomes as well as the translocation of genes from one chromosome to another produce all varieties of abnormalities in the synapsis of the chromosomes in the germ cells as well as the synapsis of the giant chromosomes in the salivary gland. On this account, the cross-breeding of even closely related varieties, such as these two flies, gives rise to hybrid offspring that are themselves perfectly sterile and unable to bring about a normal reduction in their chromosomal number. The two varieties of Drosophila have no doubt been derived from a common ancestor, but the series of mutations which has occurred in one of them has been quite different from the genic mutations which have taken place in the other. Isolation and separation of individuals in geographic range and in other environmental ways may tend to differentiate groups simply through the occurrence of different spontaneous mutations which may possibly be entirely independent of environmental differences to which the groups are subjected. The problem of the genetics of a population as a whole is not exactly the same as that of the genetics of the individual.

THE GENE IN BACTERIA AND DISEASE VIRUSES

A number of questions finally suggest themselves: if genes are more or less independent units or entities need they necessarily be grouped together to form chromosomes? Are genes capable of separate and independent existence, or have they undergone evolution of their arrangement from free separate entities into a final dependence upon a grouping into chromosomes? Such questions lead us to think of those things in nature other than animals and plants which also are capable of increasing their kind and of producing more material like unto themselves. Bacteria are not typical cells since they have no discreet nucleus as do the cells of plants and animals. Yet the bacterium possesses small chromatin-like granules scattered throughout its substance. Bacteria multiply themselves and also mutate and change. May not the granules in their substance be small groups of genes or single large genes not yet arranged into chromosomes? The origin of the cell-nucleus might only be possible after the genes have alined themselves into chromosomes and thus the bacterium lacks a nucleus. But the gene-like particles in the bacterium may be the forerunner of a nucleus and may be the stuff giving rise to its activities as well as differentiating one type of bacterium from another. Disease causing bacteria may give off substances produced by the action of their genes which alter the normal conditions under which the genes of the host cells tend to be maintained. The struggle between the host and the bacterial infection may be perchance a combat between the states induced by antagonistic genes. In certain cases the host finally overcomes the bacteria by an environmental reaction unfavorable to their existence. The host is free of the bacteria and may permanently retain a modified condition rendering it now unfavorable for this bacterium; we call this immunity. If immune reactions involve such organic particles as the genes, we may readily imagine a means for the inheritance of immunities in certain cases. Possibly genic mutations themselves may at times arise as responses to certain bacterial genes.

Assuming the constitution of bacteria to be due to the presence of separate and unarranged genes in their substratum, we may theorize a step further and imagine the possibility of the independent existence of single gene stuff. The independent gene would need to have no definable attribute of life except the power to reproduce from the limited environment other molecules like itself. Such a molecule might fill the rôle of a disease-causing virus. This virus can increase in amount or reproduce itself only in certain hosts or environments. The presence of this independent gene or virus within the cells of a host might disturb the function of particular host genes and cause disease reactions. Independent genes, if such exist, may be only single organic molecules and might lend themselves to isolation in pure crystalline form in the same way as Stanley of the Rockefeller Institute has found for the virus of tobacco-mosaic disease. We may imagine again a reaction in the host towards these free genes or viruses which brings about either temporary recovery or permanent immunity from the disease-producing effects.

Such theories must be taken seriously since if bacteria are living organisms, genes certainly are concerned in their constitution. Also the ultimate life-molecule would need only to possess the power of self-synthesis and possible contact effects on other molecules to fulfil the behavior of both the gene and a disease virus.

The finer details of the mechanisms of heredity have been learned from studies made during the last quarter century. Many of the more fundamental and far-reaching of these studies have originated in this country, chiefly by T. H. Morgan and his school of workers. Important problems still remain. No one yet knows how a gene multiplies itself causing its prototype to reappear in the millions of body cells derived from the original egg which contained only a single gene of the kind. Is the gene the ultimate unit which possesses that marvelous property characteristic of the molecules of living stuff: the ability to self-synthesize from the environment and produce other entities identically the same as itself?

No one knows how genes act in stimulating differentiation during embryonic development to finally bring about the characters of the adult. How do genes influence the quality of cells causing those in one group to differ from those of another although each cell contains the same complement of genes? Does the specifically differentiated cytoplasm of each body tissue and organ interact with the genes?

There should be found some connection between the genes and the organizing substances which Spemann's recent work has so greatly elucidated. The way in which the genes bring about a specific type of development is almost completely unknown.

III

MEDICINE AT SEA IN THE DAYS OF SAIL

BY

KARL VOGEL, M.D.

ASSOCIATE PROFESSOR OF CLINICAL PATHOLOGY,
COLLEGE OF PHYSICIANS AND SURGEONS, COLUMBIA UNIVERSITY

III

MEDICINE AT SEA IN THE DAYS OF SAIL

THE professional students of human behavior—those enviable persons whose agreeable occupation it is to reflect upon the weaknesses and hidden motives of other people—sometimes apply to certain quite admirable kinds of reading matter the slightly supercilious designation of "escape literature." The fairy tales of childhood, the cowboy and Tarzan thrillers of adolescence, and the murder mysteries and "boy-meets-girl" fiction of maturer years, all open the portals into a bright world of make-believe in which cares are momentarily forgotten and we can grow in self-importance by subconsciously identifying ourselves with imaginary heroes—supermen and women of surpassing strength, intelligence, and beauty. The sagas of the sea, authentic or fictitious, rank high in the category of such emollients to harassed egos. There are few who do not feel the appeal of these fascinating narratives of adventurers lured by legends of Cathay and Eldorado, of coral islands lapped by azure seas, or of bloody fights on black and rakish pirate luggers, aboard which lovely señoritas by the narrowest of margins escape a fate reputed to be worse than death.

It seems a pity to dim the colors of these romantic

fancies, but as a matter of fact their actual background was pretty drab and grim. Life at sea in the early days of sail was hideously uncomfortable, and the magnificent hardihood of those who braved it was only too often inspired by nothing more praiseworthy than the profit motive—the hope of riches to be gained by trade, or by the more brutal outrages of plunder and depredation. Even the glamour of the great voyage of Columbus loses a little of its luster when we remember that it was a purely business venture, undertaken on a contingent basis of 10 per cent of the proceeds. The astounding courage of the conquistadores was animated by the greed for gold, and though they attempted and achieved the impossible, and poured untold treasure into the coffers of their country, it was at the expense of savage cruelty and injustice to unoffending native races that were enslaved and exterminated. The Elizabethan sea-dogs were actuated by hatred of the Spaniard and envy of his wealth, so they raided and burned his young settlements in the New World, and plundered the stately galleons wallowing into Acapulco heavy with the riches extorted from the Philippines or Peru. In the days when refrigeration was still unknown, food quickly spoiled, and to mitigate its rankness pepper, cloves, cinnamon, nutmeg, mace, and other condiments were valued to a degree that we can hardly realize. The overland journey to secure these and the other rich commodities of the East was long and costly, so, step by step, Africa was circumnavigated and the frigid regions of the Arctic were explored, in the hope of greater profits by finding a cheaper route to the fragrant islands whence came the spices, and the no less highly prized gums and balsams necessary to the medicine of that time.

One cannot get a better idea of what his life seemed like to the early sailor than from a remarkable seventeenth-century manuscript which has only recently come to light and been transcribed from the original by Basil Lubbock. It is the journal, hundreds of pages long and most engaging in its phraseology, kept for many years by an ordinary seaman, Edward Barlow by name. As a detailed chronicle of the daily doings of a humbler individual of exactly the same period it forms a fitting pendant to Samuel Pepys' immortal record of self-revelation, which also was largely concerned with nautical affairs, though chiefly from the administrative side.

On his way to "Lisborne" in 1661, food and water ran short, and Barlow says:

> We were now forced to go to one quart of "befraiage" to one man a day, which "befraiage" was made of sour wine and stinking water, which was very hard with us; and the weather being hot and always eating salt victuals, I could not get my belly full, which made me often repent of my going to sea.... And I was always thinking that beggars had a far better life of it and lived better than I did, for they seldom missed of their bellies full of better victuals than we could get; and also at night to lie quiet and out of danger in a good barn full of straw, nobody disturbing them and might lie as long as they pleased; but it was quite contrary with us, for we seldom in a month got our belly full of victuals,

and that of such salt as many beggars would think scorn to eat; and at night when we went to take our rest, we were not to lie still above four hours; and many times when it blew hard we were not sure to lie one hour, yea often we were called up before we had slept one half hour and forced to go up into the main top or the fore top to take in our topsails, half awake and half asleep, with one shoe on and the other shoe off, not having time to put it on; always sleeping in our clothes for readiness; and in stormy weather when the ship rolled and tumbled as though some great millstone were rolling up one hill and down another we had much ado to hold ourselves fast by the small ropes from falling by the board; and being gotten up into the tops there we must haul and pull to make fast the sail, seeing nothing but air above us and water beneath us, and that so raging as though every wave would make a grave for us; and many times the nights so dark we could not see one another, and blowing so hard that we could not hear one another speak, being close to one another; and thundering and lightening as though Heaven and earth would come together, it being usual in those countries, with showers of rain so hard it will wet a man "dunge wet" before he can go the length of the ship.

In the "spacious days" of Queen Elizabeth, when Drake, Raleigh, Hawkins, Frobisher, Gilbert, and the others were roaming and raiding the world in her service, the treatment of the sailors was inhumanly bad, and the crews that singed the Spanish King's beard by smashing the Invincible Armada, the proudest fleet the world till then had seen, were wretchedly clothed, half-starved, and riddled with infection. Under the Stuarts conditions were no better, and just seven years after the *Mayflower* had sailed from Plymouth we find Admiral Mervyn writing to Buckingham that the seamen were sickening so fast that the King would shortly have more ships than men, and lamenting:

> ... the more than miserable condition of the men, who have neither shoes, stockings nor rags to cover their nakedness. All the ships are so infectious that I fear if we hold the sea one month we shall not bring enough men home to moor the ships. You may think I make it worse, but I vow to God I cannot deliver it in words. ... The poor men bear all as patiently as they can.... I much wonder that so little care be taken to preserve men that are so hardly bred. I have used my best cunning to make the *Vanguard* wholesome. I have caused her to be washed all over, fore and aft, every second day; to be perfumed with tar burnt and frankincense; to be aired twixt decks with pans of charcoal; to be twice a week washed with vinegar.... Yet if today we get together two hundred men within four days afterwards we have not one hundred.

The ships of that time were resplendent with gilded carving and streamed silken banners from every spar, but there was no thought for the sick or wounded sailor. When the ship went into action he was bundled out of the way into the dank and dismal cable tier or was stretched on the foul and stinking ballast. If he survived the medical science of the day and was landed disabled there was little or no provision for his care, though in 1590 a sort of mutual benefit fund called the Chatham Chest was established and supported by taking sixpence a month from the meager pay of every man and boy in the navy. There was a further deduction of twopence for the ship's surgeon, but the health of the soul was seemingly esteemed twice as highly as that of the body for double this amount was abstracted for the benefit of the chaplain. It was not until the Commonwealth that there were any effective measures for looking after the sick and wounded; hospital ships were added to the fleet, naval hospitals were founded on shore, and the beginning of a pension system was instituted.

Overcrowding and bad food were the great sources of disease and operated in a vicious circle. The complement of the famous *Henri Grace à Dieu* of Henry VIII which was about the size of an American thirty-six gun frigate, was seven hundred men or more, and the *Mary Rose* of the same period, a vessel of only six hundred tons, had five or six hundred men crowded into her. Some centuries later crews of three hundred, and one hundred and eighty respectively would have been considered correct for ships of this size. Much larger numbers were sometimes carried, as on the *Great Michael* of 1514, which is credited with a force composed of a thousand fighting men, one hundred and twenty gunners, and three hundred mariners—over fourteen hundred in all; and a French ship *Marie la Cordelière* is stated to have been manned by from fifteen hundred to two thousand men, soldiers and sailors.

The diet was so restricted in variety and so deficient in the essentials for well-balanced nutrition that it is no wonder scurvy and other diseases were so prevalent. The regulation ration for the middle of the seventeenth century was as follows: In addition to a gallon of beer and a pound of biscuit daily, on Sundays and Tuesdays two pounds of salt beef; on Mondays and Thursdays one pound of salt pork and one pint of peas, or if pork was lacking one pound and a half of beef instead; on Wednesdays, Fridays and Saturdays one-eighth part of a "sized" fish, one-eighth of a pound of butter and one quarter of a pound of cheese. The standard fish sizes were twenty-four inches for cod, twenty-two inches for haberdine, and a one-half-sized stock fish was supposed to measure sixteen inches. Even more serious than the limited variety of the foodstuffs was the fact that through imperfect means of preservation and the outrageous dishonesty of the contractors they were nearly always more or less decomposed and wholly unfit for human consumption, but if condemned and returned they were often enough repacked and sent to other ships. A contemporary commentator remarks: "I must needs say that here hath been found very ill dealing; and that not only in the provision of flesh . . . but in the rottenness of the cheese, in the frowsiness and foul condition of the butter, and in the badness of the salted fish . . . and as for the beer it was for the most part very undrinkable."

In the merchant service where the individual commander had some discretion and authority the conditions were not necessarily so bad. Captain Luke Foxe of Hull was one of the long list of those who sought fame and fortune by attempting to tap the treasures of the East by way of the icy northwest passage, and was evidently quite pleased with the superior quality of his commissariat, and also of his medical supplies, for he records that when he set out in 1631 he

> ...was victualled compleatly for 18 moneths.... I had excellent fat Beefe, strong Beere, good wheaten Bread, good Island Ling, Butter and Cheese of the best, admirable Sacke and Aqua Vitae, Pease, Oat-meale, Wheatmeale, Oyle, Spice, Suger, Fruit and Rice, with Chyrurgerie, as Sirrups, Iulips, Condits, Trechissis, antidotes, balsoms, gummes, unguents, implaisters, oyles, potions, suppositors, and purging Pils; and if I had wanted Instruments, my Chyrurgion had enough.

Salt beef and pork, green and moldy, and hardtack crawling with weevils remained the staples of the seaman's nutriment until comparatively recent times, and even our frigates of the War of 1812 were fitted out with only the following provisions: Beef, pork, molasses, rice, butter, cheese, vinegar, beans, rum, flour, Indian meal, bread, potatoes, and salt fish.

While this absence of regard for the well-being and medical care of the seaman seems to-day appalling and inexcusable, it must be remembered that his contemporaries on shore, even the most highly placed, were not very happily situated either in regard to health conditions, and it has been stated that during the thirteenth century people of sixty-five were not as frequently seen as those of eighty are to-day. Indeed, the surgeon of one hospital ship, the *Jeffries,* in commission in 1700, made the claim, "We lose not so many in proportion as candid physicians in London own, viz., one out of every five sick, and think that they come off well to boot."

Many generations of human beings had to suffer

misery, pain, and early death before the medical infant became vigorous enough to throw off the swaddling clothes in which the doctrines and authority of Galen had swathed it fourteen centuries earlier. Finally the Hippocratic method of clinical observation and common sense began to supersede the blind and unreasoning adherence to tradition with which the successors of Galen, through all the intervening years, had smothered any semblance of effective progress, and medicine too, much more tardily than culture in general, entered into its renaissance.

At about the period of our Revolution three naval surgeons, James Lind, Thomas Trotter, and Sir Gilbert Blane, and also the famous explorer Captain James Cook, changed the whole complexion of the seaman's life by introducing reforms that were so important and so beneficial that the names of these great sanitarians should be written high in every hall of fame. Scurvy, due to the faulty diet, deficient as we now understand in vitamins, was conquered by Lind's demonstration of the value of fresh vegetables and especially the citrus fruits, a doctrine long known but till then never consistently applied. The frightful epidemics of typhus and typhoid—then significantly called ship fever or gaol fever—smallpox, tropical fevers or calentures, and dysentery or the bloody flux, were greatly reduced by the enforcement of systematic regulations making for cleanliness and general sanitation. Methods of ventilation were devised, newly drafted men were medically examined and scrubbed before they were allowed to enter healthy ships, soap was issued to the crews and they were obliged to keep their bodies and clothing clean. A space on each ship called the sick bay was set aside for hospital purposes, though originally its location was not definite and varied according to the convenience of the moment. In 1800 at the instance of Lord St. Vincent the Admiralty ordered that no sick were to be kept below the upper deck of any line-of-battle ship, and that the sick berth was to be established under the forecastle on the starboard side with a roundhouse [latrine] enclosed for the use of the invalids. Ambulant patients were treated at regular clinics held twice a day at the foremast by the assistant surgeons and their stewards or loblolly boys. By way of contrast to the severe discipline and savage floggings that were so frequent it is a truly pleasant thing to read of the consideration the captain and other officers appear to have shown in contributing from their tables whatever was available in the way of wines, fresh meat, or other additions to the regular ship's supplies for those in the sick bay. Captain Basil Hall states that after the carver in the gun-room has helped his messmates he generally turns to the surgeon and says: "Doctor, what shall I send to the sick?"

Scurvy was the greatest single enemy of the early seaman and nearly always was present to some extent on ships engaged in long voyages. Its symptoms were horrible and loathsome, particularly under the existing conditions where no nursing care was possible, as may be seen from the typical description given by William Hutchinson, later a famous captain, who endured its miseries for three months while serving as a forecastle man in a ship on its way to the East Indies in 1738. After a gradual onset of increasing weakness which finally become so extreme that he lost the use of his hands and feet so that he could not even crawl up the ladder to the deck he says:

> I thus struggled with the disease 'till it increased so that my armpits and hams grew black, and I pined away to a weak helpless condition, with my teeth all loose, and my upper and lower gums swelled and clotted together like a jelly, and they bled to that degree that I was obliged to lie with my mouth hanging over the side of my hammock, to let the blood run out and to keep it from clotting so as to choak me; 'till after a seven months passage we arrived in Pullicat Road; from whence we got fresh provisions, and sent for men to carry the ship to Madras, where what remained of the sick were got on shore to sick quarters; and where with fresh provisions and fomentations of herbs I got well and returned on board in eighteen days.

During an engagement the decks were sanded to make them less slippery from blood, and the petty officers and many of the men themselves carried tourniquets with which to check the hemorrhage from limbs shattered by shot or caused by the even more ghastly injuries due to flying splinters. The hopelessly wounded were thrown overboard at once, otherwise the victim had to make his way or be assisted by his messmates down the steep ladders to the cockpit, a dark space below the waterline, normally the midshipmen's berth but now used as an operating room. Here by dim lantern light the surgeon and his mates took each man rigidly in his turn, working at top speed on patients whose courage—with a tot of rum—was their only anesthetic. Conservative surgery was unknown, and would have been impossible. An arm or leg, if a hasty inspection showed that it was at all badly wounded was amputated as a matter of course—for abdominal and thoracic injuries little could be done except to probe for foreign bodies and apply a dressing. Skull fractures were trephined and usually ended in brain abscess. Tetanus and infection were responsible for many deaths, but the ultimate results following even dreadfully severe operations were sometimes surprisingly good. William Burd, Surgeon of the *Niger,* gives a detailed account of an amputation at the shoulder joint for a compound comminuted gunshot fracture of the head of the humerus, performed at sea, which is harrowing to read, for one cannot forget that it was done on a fully conscious patient. The assisting French surgeon, a prisoner of war, whose responsibility it was to control the subclavian artery by digital compression lost his nerve, and as Burd says "forsook him" at the most critical moment, but Burd succeeded in completing the operation "without the loss of so much blood as might have been expected," and three and a half months later the patient was discharged perfectly well.

Incongruous as it seems, lack of fresh air, or perhaps better said, the presence of extremely foul air, was responsible for much discomfort and disease on shipboard. It might appear that the one place above all others where one would be sure to enjoy the pure breath of heaven most abundantly would be on a sailing ship in the middle of the ocean, and it is true that while he remained on deck the sailor had plenty of it, and often indeed too much, but as soon as he stepped below he entered an atmosphere usually either too cold and too damp or too hot and too damp, and always sickeningly offensive to the sense of smell. The latter quality was sometimes developed to an extreme point, and it has been stated, for example, that in 1739 the ships in the squadron anchored at Spithead "stunk to such a degree" that they infected each other and the men became so dangerously ill that they had to be put ashore. Lind gives a description of the conditions on the *Panther* which reveals what an abode of misery and generator of stenches the sick bay could be. During the voyage home forty men died of scurvy and there were usually ninety patients huddled in a place with no provision whatever for ventilation. The atmosphere was so suffocating that the sick were stifled for want of air, and the surgeon when visiting them could hardly breathe or remain for any length of time without going often on deck, or reviving himself with spirit of hartshorn or a glass of wine. The dampness was particularly bad in new vessels for the timber was often unseasoned or had been treated with brine to make it more durable, and it took many months before they dried out and were free from mildew. Large ships were worse in this respect than small, and some were notoriously bad, like the *Arrogant,* of which it was said that the decks and beams were remarkable for their moisture which seemed to exhale from the timbers, and one of her officers has noted that he "observed the damp vapor on his bed-cloaths every morning like a heavy dew." In addition there was the moisture produced by the wet clothing of the men which in bad weather never had a chance to dry, and to make matters still worse there was the routine flooding of the decks. A passion for snowy decks has ever been an obsession with executive officers, and seamen of all ages have had to suffer the affliction of holystoning. The scrubbing and the sluicing of the lower decks with water was particularly objectionable if done after sunset so that they remained wet for hours, and many surgeons protested against this practice. Some officers advocated dry holystoning, which obviated the floods of water but filled the air with dust.

Hundreds of unwashed men had to sleep so crowded together that their hammocks touched—fourteen to eighteen inches was the regulation space for each—and the sick bay contributed its share of noisomeness, particularly after an engagement when there would be many infected wounds, or if there was an epidemic on board. The ballast was likely to be wet and malodorous, and the bilges reeked with stagnant and polluted water which generated gases so noxious that when the ship's well was to be cleaned a lighted candle had to be lowered first to see if it was safe for a man to enter without danger of asphyxiation. The earlier efforts at ventilation were limited to the use of wind sails, great conical tubes of canvas intended to convey a current of fresh air down the hatches, and the occasional resort to fires in pots or small stoves that were moved from place to place to create an upward draft and to dry out the ship. Really effective measures were not developed until the middle of the eighteenth century when various types of windmills and other mechanical ventilators were introduced. One form which acted like gigantic bellows was invented by a clergyman, Dr. Hales, and continued in use for over fifty years. The improvement in health that followed was remarkable, and the Earl of Halifax is credited with the statement that for every twelve men dying on unventilated ships there was but one death on those which used the new appliances.

A favorite sanitary measure was washing the inside of the ship with boiling vinegar; but the greatest reliance was placed on fumigation. For this purpose everything seems to have been used that could make a bad smell—pitch, brimstone, tarry old rope, condemned tobacco, tar, charcoal, asafetida, niter, or common salt mixed with vitriolic acid, and gunpowder dampened with vinegar. This was also sometimes flashed from pistols, on the theory that the shock of the explosion would "disperse the infectious matter from the timbers of the ship." Vinegar was vaporized by plunging a red-hot loggerhead or an iron ball into a bucketful, or by heating over a lamp. Trotter was not much impressed by a special device designed for the latter use, saying that "the smell of the vapor is very agreeable but I would say no more for it. It ought to be trusted, like lavender water on the handkerchief of a belle or a beau."

Providing a sufficient supply of drinking water and keeping it in usable condition has always been one of the major problems on long voyages. Commonly of unsatisfactory quality to begin with and stored in wooden casks, it soon became foul; was often the cause of epidemics, and complaints regarding it are frequent, long, and loud: "The water so putrid, thick and stinking that often I have held my nose with my hand while I drank it strained through my pocket handkerchief, and we were so short of this necessary article that our consumption was limited to two pints a day for all purposes." This was not the wail of a disgruntled foremast hand but was written by an Admiral of the British Navy, in referring to a time as comparatively recent as the Trafalgar period.

To prevent the slimy vegetable growth that coated the inside of the casks and pervaded the water different expedients were resorted to, such as charring the casks, soaking them first in sea water, or adding various preservatives. Among these were alum and cream of tartar, but the most widely used was quicklime in the proportion of about a pound to each water butt. This was effective in preventing putrefaction but added a disagreeable taste and unpleasant quality, though one medical writer says that it was not injurious to health, but "on the contrary friendly to the bowels." Still, various procedures were suggested to precipitate the lime before use, such as by the addition of magnesia, which was too expensive, or by devices for generating carbon dioxide in the cask, which were much too complicated for use on shipboard. Another method of sweetening offensive water was by means of an apparatus invented by Lieutenant Osbridge of the British Navy. The water was raised several feet by a pump fixed to the scuttle butt and then caused to be exposed to the air in a finely divided state by being allowed to fall through a series of perforated metal disks placed horizontally at intervals in a long cylinder. This worked very well, and Trotter says that no ship should go to sea without it.

It was not until the early part of the last century that the whole difficulty was solved very simply by the substitution of iron tanks for the wooden casks. The matter was discussed in a report on the health of the British Navy published in 1841, and it was stated that:

When water was kept in wooden casks it became slightly foetid from the disengagement of hydrogen in a few days, and in a fortnight or three weeks so loathsome as to be swallowed with repugnance, even when called for by urgent thirst. The progress of decomposition and its nauseating results were especially rapid and offensive when the water was most pure, at least when it contained the smallest proportion of mineral admixture and the temperature was high. When the solid food consisted almost exclusively of very salt beef and pork, biscuits long baked, and puddings made of salt, suet, and flour, the desire for—even the necessity of—abundance of water was great. No one who has not felt it can imagine the distress that was often endured within the tropics, setting aside the effects on health, from the intense thirst thus excited, and the only means available for quenching it water so putrid and offensive, often so thick and green from vegetable admixture and decomposition, and emitting so strongly the foetor of rotten eggs as to disgust at once the sense of smell and taste.

In iron tanks the water kept indefinitely without alteration. The change from wooden to iron containers was begun shortly after the turn of the century and after it had been effected throughout the service there was a great improvement in the seamen's health.

A hundred years ago in the British Navy the amount of water issued was left to the discretion of the captain, but it was customary to allow each man an Imperial gallon, including what was needed for cooking and for mixing grog. In the American Navy the official allowance was less, the regulations stipulating at least one-half gallon per man on foreign voyages, and more on the Home Station, but the captain was authorized to shorten this allowance if desirable. An interesting order has been preserved, issued by Captain Thomas Truxton of the frigate *Constellation* in 1798, showing the routine in use at that time:

ON BOARD THE *Constellation*

Order for the Preservation of Health, and Care of Water, to commence on the 29th of June 1798—

At seven Bells, or at half past seven o'clock every Morning, the Crew is to be served one Pint of Water. at half an Hour before Noon, one Pint of Grog.— At half past 3 in the Afternoon, another Pint of Grog; at half an Hour before Sun Set every Evening they are to have served them a Pint and a half a Pint of Water, making in the whole four Pints, and half a Pint of Water, and half a Pint of Rum, which is mixed as aforesaid.—

This is the Allowance of Rum and Water,—(Exclusive of that for boiling Pease) for Twenty four hours, under existing Circumstances, and is to continue, untill further Orders from me in Writing.

In serving out the Water, each Man may be allowed, to take his Allowance with him, provided he has Anything to put in it, those who have not, must have it put in the Scuttle Cask, under a Centinel who is to guard the same with a Cutlass; as no Muskets are suffered on Deck at Sea, but when at Quarters.—

N. B. No more Water is to be allowed for my use, than for any other Man—without a Special Order, two Quarts per Day excepted for the Use of Officers at my Table.—

THOMAS TRUXTUN

To The Sea Leiutenants and Master &C.

Owing to the difficulty of keeping water in a drinkable condition, for centuries the traditional beverage of the sailor was beer, and it was customary to say that bread, beef, and beer were the backbone of the British Navy. The allowance was the handsome amount of a gallon a day, but through the dishonesty of grafting contractors it was often miserable in quality and speedily spoiled, so that epidemics of intestinal disorders were common and the frightful mortality from disease on the ships of Elizabeth and her successors is supposed to have been in large part due to this cause. Lord Howard of Effingham, the Admiral in command of the fleet that defeated the Spanish Armada, protested that though the beer had been condemned as unfit for use it was still being issued to the men, and added the rather mild comment that "nothing doth displease the seamen more than sour beer." Their displeasure must have been further increased if it was true as Sir Walter Raleigh complained, that often it was kept in casks that had previously been used for oil or fish. The evil was perennial, for a hundred and fifty years later we find Admiral Hawke whose fleet was blockading Brest sending to the official at Plymouth who was responsible for supplies the terse admonition: "The beer brewed at your port is so excessively bad that it employs the whole time of the squadron in surveying it and throwing it overboard."

In later times wine or spirits were substituted for the beer, a pint of the former or one half pint of rum or brandy being issued in its place. The earlier practice of serving rum undiluted was found to have its drawbacks, and it became the custom to mix it with three or four parts of water before giving it to the men, usually in two daily portions. This improvement is due to Admiral Vernon, who in 1740 called for a report on the matter from his captains and surgeons and then put in force their unanimous recommendation that the rum be watered. Unexpected manifestations of human ingenuity are often quite delightful, and there was a rather pleasing directness in the habit of choosing the men designated to serve the beverage from the size of their thumbs. This was because in doling out the precious balm the thirsty sailor's cup was most advantageously grasped with the outstretched thumb inside, and the amount saved by this short measurement went to swell the residue which was the perquisite of those in charge of the distribution. The admiral was known to the sailors as Old Grog because of the huge cloak of grogram cloth he used to sport in stormy weather, and his invention has been called grog ever since. In the American Navy the rum allowance originally was also one half pint, and the frigates that won the victories of 1812 were provided with the impressive amount of eight thousand five hundred gallons of the cheering fluid when setting out on a twelvemonth's cruise. Existing figures of the cost of fitting out a vessel of this type show that the yearly estimate for all the provisions was a little over twenty-eight thousand dollars, and as the rum was quoted at one dollar a gallon the outlay for this one item made up not far from one third of the entire sum. It is instructive to note that the corresponding figure for all medical and surgical supplies was only two thousand five hundred dollars. At a subsequent period the rum ration was reduced to one gill and during the Civil War it was discontinued entirely. By many commanders and most naval surgeons the issue of the large allowance of spirits was considered prejudicial to discipline and health, and Trotter even went so far as to say that the treatment of intoxication was the most frequent part of the surgeon's duty, but though the punishments for drunkenness were severe the seaman considered his grog the most important compensation for his many hardships. One tot was not enough to make much of an impression on a tough old salt, but by saving up his allowance and perhaps adding to it other portions secured by fair means or foul from his messmates he could on occasion get himself into a state of most satisfactory cheerfulness.

In the mercantile marine of later times the captain with the aid of the ship's medicine chest had to fulfil the functions of physician and surgeon, and sometimes of accoucheur as well, in addition to his more strictly nautical duties. With the well-known ingenuity of the sailor, and thanks to the force of character which alone could make it possible for him to maintain his position as the supreme ruler of his little floating world, the emergencies that arose seem to have been dealt with fairly well. The masters of sailing ships were often astonishingly young and one cannot but wonder at the self-reliance with which they faced their complex responsibilities. Captain Nathaniel Brown Palmer was only twenty-one when in 1821 he took the tiny sealing sloop *Hero* from Stonington to the Antarctic and was the first to explore the region known by his name until later cartographers changed it to Graham Land, and Captain Isaiah West of New Bedford commanded a whaler at twenty-two. A well-known surgeon has told me of an incident early in the career of his father, who after a life of active seafaring is still in good health in his home in Scotland at the age of eighty-four. When only twenty-three, while in Calcutta, he was appointed first mate of the *Indian Empire,* a full-rigged ship of two thousand tons. Soon after sailing the captain who had long been ailing died, and the young mate succeeded to the command. Some of the tanks had been filled with tainted water so that an outbreak of cholera developed on board, but in spite of the fact that a large proportion of the crew were disabled and eight of them succumbed to the disease, the youthful captain brought his ship safely home to Dundee. Imagine his anxiety as sailor after sailor sickened and he wondered when, if ever, the pestilence would cease. One is reminded of Joseph Conrad's trials when he received his first command, described by him as fiction in one of his finest stories, but actually based on his own experience. Appointed to the bark *Otago* to replace the captain who had died at sea, he set sail from Bangkok for Melbourne, the ship was becalmed in the torrid gulf of Siam, and the crew began to come down with tropical malaria until all except Conrad and the ship's cook were incapacitated. Then came the calamity of discovering that the former captain who apparently was of unsound mind had disposed of the reserve stock of quinine which should have been in the medicine chest, and refilled the bottles with an inert substitute. Nevertheless, Conrad succeeded in working the ship, filled with helpless invalids, as far as Singapore, where he shipped a new crew and then completed the voyage to Australia.

A chapter of sailing-ship history that remains to be written concerns the heroism of the women on shipboard who sometimes in addition to the perils of the sea willingly faced those of bringing a child into the world with no possibility of medical aid. British captains, as well as those aristocrats of the ocean the New England skippers, not infrequently took their wives with them on long voyages, often as the only woman on board. A friend of mine, Captain B—— first saw the light of day off the Horn, and every one of his five brothers and sisters was also born at sea in widely different parts of the globe. He is of the fourth generation of a famous line of Maine shipmasters and was only nineteen when he was made captain of the *Herbert Black* of Searsport, and at twenty-three was given command of the *Bangalore,* a splendidly built fifteen-hundred-ton three skysail ship engaged in the Australian and Hawaiian trade. During his days at sea his medical and surgical experiences were many and various and calculated to tax the resources of a trained medical man, such as saving the life of his mate after fourteen days of intestinal obstruction and successfully conducting a confinement during the height of a violent gale. His brother who had preceded him in the command of the *Herbert Black,* a small bark of five hundred and fifty-four tons, was only twenty-five when in that vessel he performed a feat of seamanship such as has seldom been equaled. While rounding the Horn his rudder was lost, but he managed to construct and ship a substitute, getting his material by cutting up a spare topmast. At that time beriberi was common on ships touching the west coast of South and Central America; the disease appeared on board and his mate, second mate, and four of the eight remaining members of the crew died of it. In spite of this he navigated his leaking ship with a jury rudder and a sick and dying crew to Barbados, the few left alive so weakened that on his arrival there help had to be summoned from shore to take the sail off the ship.

The ship's medicine chest usually included a booklet of instructions, and sometimes to simplify the difficult arts of diagnosis and treatment different diseases were numbered to correspond with the bottles containing suitable remedies in each case. A favorite tale, perhaps as apocryphal as most salt-water yarns, is of an ingenious captain, who having decided that his patient presented symptom complex No. 9 and finding this bottle empty, rose to the situation by administering equal doses of No. 3 and No. 6. Most of the time the problems were not difficult. Job-like the sailor is a martyr to boils and these were the commonest surgical condition, while constipation was the most prevalent medical complaint, but was kept in subjection by the enormous quantities of Epsom salts which formed the most important component of the stock of drugs.

These medical counselors to the captain, are often interesting and remarkable. One of them which is called *Cox's Companion to the Sea Medicine Chest* seems to have been a great favorite for it had already run through thirty-three editions in England when it was published in New York in 1851. It must have presented the baffled amateur practitioner with a rather mystifying array of therapeutic possibilities, for it belongs to the machine-gun era of prescribing and about two hundred different drugs are discussed. Many of these are herbs or other vegetable remedies with such animalistic names as snake-root, worm-grass, skunk-cabbage, cranesbill, cowhage, bearberry, dogwood, and dozens of others that have long since passed into the limbo of forgotten things. Several pages are devoted to the resuscitation of the apparently drowned, chief reliance being placed on insufflation of the lungs with bellows, either through the nostril or preferably by passing a curved tin tube attached to the nozzle into the patient's larynx, a feat that if successfully performed would command sincerest admiration. Two life-giving procedures warmly recommended by earlier authorities had apparently been discarded by this time for they are not mentioned. One consisted in having the operator apply his mouth to that of the patient and so blow air into his lungs—if he first chewed garlic the effect was considered to be more reviving—and the other was the introduction of tobacco smoke into the bowel. A generation later another book which also ran through many editions was *The Ship Captain's Medical Guide,* and as its author Dr. Leach, was Physician to the Dreadnought Seaman's Hospital of London it is thoroughly practical and the treatments and other procedures advised are not beyond the resources or abilities of the average ship's officer. It is somewhat remarkable, however, that although there is a good deal of matter relating to the management of venereal diseases, which are said to be "the bane of the mercantile marine service," there is not one single word of warning about the necessity of taking precautions to prevent the transmission of infection to others. A *Handbook for the Ship's Medicine Chest* prepared under the auspices of the United States Marine Hospital Service was—and still is—widely circulated in the American merchant marine. This is a wholly admirable manual, and the 1900 edition issued while sailing ships were still making long voyages gives well-selected lists of medicines and drugs, and is written with regard to simplicity in medication and due emphasis on antisepsis and the prevention of contagion.

Shortly after the War of 1812 had demonstrated the efficiency of the American Navy a new phase developed in maritime history which gave the young republic a supremacy on the Atlantic which was to endure for many years. The lure of the new land of promise attracted the enterprising or the discontented of the Old World and an ever-increasing stream of emigration began to cross the ocean. To meet this demand, in 1816, the Black Ball Line of packet ships was established, soon followed by numerous others, and these Western Ocean Packets as they were called rapidly acquired the domination of the passenger trade between English and American ports. While the Continent contributed its share, the majority of the emigrants at this time were English, Irish, and Scottish, and the records show that between 1815 and 1854 over four million passengers left the British Isles, and of these nearly two and a half million sailed during the eight years preceding the latter date. The earlier packet ships were small, of about five hundred tons, but as the traffic grew they increased in capacity up to three times that size or more, but all designed for speed, heavily sparred, and well adapted to cope with the gales of the North Atlantic. Beating against the prevailing westerlies was slow work, and the average passage to the States took forty days. In the other direction better time was possible, the average being twenty-three days, but phenomenally quick crossings were not infrequent and several records of less than fourteen days are well authenticated. These were the halcyon days of sail, and though steamship lines began to be established about 1840, for many years the swift sailing-ships not infrequently made better passages than the power-driven vessels. When Charles Dickens astonished the literary world by visiting this country in 1842 he came in the Cunarder *Britannia,* but for the return journey he chose the sailing packet *George Washington* and had the satisfaction of arriving a day ahead of the steamer. In his *American Notes* he gives a lengthy and vivid description of the discomforts of ocean travel in those days, and later utilized his experiences in depicting Martin Chuzzlewit's journey in the steerage of a packet ship, where the miseries of the emigrants almost broke down the optimism of even the incurably cheerful Mark Tapley.

Lubbock quotes an old packet captain as having written:

> Men, women and children were tumbled into the 'tween decks together, dirty, saucy, ignorant and breed-

ing the most loathsome of creeping things. The stench below decks, aggravated by the seasickness and the ship's poor equipment for the work, placed us far below the civilization of the dark ages. It was not uncommon in mid-winter to be fifty or sixty days making the homeward passage. In gales, which were frequent, hatches had to be battened down and men, women and children screamed all night in terror. Ship fever, smallpox, and other diseases were common, and it is a wonder that so many survived the voyage as really did.

The passage rates fluctuated somewhat from year to year. In 1842 they were five pounds, but in 1851 when the emigrant traffic was at its height they fell to three pounds ten shillings from Liverpool to New York, and even less to Quebec. This comprised only the passage, and the passenger had to provide for all his needs except fire for cooking and drinking water, and before going aboard was obliged to show that he had an adequate supply of provisions. On the Black X Line, for example, the requirement was a suitable amount of flour, biscuit, potatoes, tea, sugar and treacle, two hams, a tin pot, frying-pan, mug, teapot, knife, fork, and spoon. On one of the larger vessels the space assigned to the steerage was about seventy feet long by thirty wide, with six feet between decks. Here several hundred people had to accommodate themselves in rough bunks of unplaned lumber, six feet wide divided by partitions into three sleeping places, arranged in three tiers one above the other. The alleyways, only about three feet wide, were jammed full of the piles of provisions and other belongings, over which it was necessary to crawl on all fours, and when, as was often the case during wet weather, no one was allowed on deck the crowding and lack of ventilation must have been unspeakable. Small port-holes admitted a little light but could almost never be opened and when the hatches had to be kept closed the conditions can hardly be imagined. Cooking had to be done, weather permitting, at galley fires on deck in the waist of the ship. This region was a veritable farmyard, with pens of live stock for the use of the cabin passengers, sheep, pigs, chickens, ducks, and geese, as well as cows and goats carried to supply milk, and what little space was left was reduced by the ship's long boat, spare spars and topmasts, and other nautical gear.

Under these conditions illness was inevitable and when epidemics occurred the mortality was frightful. In 1853 one ship arrived in New York with sixty cases of cholera on board, one hundred deaths having already taken place during the voyage, and eight other ships in the course of the same year reported from fifteen to eighty deaths each, and at about the same time on one vessel to the terror of an unusually rough crossing was added the horror of an outbreak of smallpox with sixty deaths. Rather oddly, it was the ship's carpenter who had charge of the emigrants, and it was his duty to keep them in order, suppress brawling, and guard against the everpresent danger of fire. When as was the case on some ships, no doctor was carried, it was he who doled out from the ship's medicine chest any remedies required and he was also the official dentist. It speaks well for the stoutness of the timber of which the American Ship of State was gradually being built that despite all these outrageous violations of every principle of sanitary science most of the steerage passengers seemed to survive, and it is stated that the births usually outnumbered the deaths. Thus it is recorded of one famous Black Ball liner, the *Independence,* that in the course of one hundred and sixteen round trips she had brought thirty thousand passengers to America, and on her decks fifteen hundred births and two hundred marriages had taken place. On some ships better provision was made for the care of the emigrants, as on the *Daniel Webster,* one of the great Donald Mackay's creations, which had iron berths on the lower deck for four hundred and fifty steerage passengers, two hospitals and a surgeon's dispensary. On her maiden voyage in 1851 she sailed from Boston to Liverpool in thirteen days, ten hours.

A highly specialized form of life at sea is represented by the whaling industry, for it was truly an industry as opposed to the carrying trade of the other branches of the mercantile marine. It was predominantly an American activity, and at the height of its development in the middle of the last century when it was estimated that the whaling fleet of the entire world numbered about nine hundred vessels, over seven hundred of these hailed from ports in the United States. Officered by men who were supreme masters of seamanship, the whale ships, slow but seaworthy, roamed the seven seas, making voyages that were measured in years, while their crews partly composed of inexperienced landsmen, led a life which E. P. Hohman says, "at its best was hard, and at its worst represented perhaps the lowest condition to which free American labor has ever fallen." Economy in operation was pushed to the utmost and the food and living conditions were commonly so bad that scurvy ravaged the forecastles of the whalers long after it had become practically extinct in all other ships. Whaling vessels of any size belonging to other nations regularly carried a surgeon, but not so in the fleets sent out from the thrifty New England towns. The risk of accidents was ever present in this the most dangerous form of big-game hunting, and stove boats, smashed by the jaws or flukes of a wounded whale, treacherous loops of flying line, or the razor edged blubber spades and knives used in the work of cutting in and trying out were the frequent cause of terrible and often fatal injuries. Any surgical aid required had to be furnished by the captain, and as surgical instruments were seldom carried he had to do the best he could with whatever means came to hand, often displaying a remarkable degree of courage and resourcefulness. These qualities were strikingly exhibited by Captain James Huntting of Southampton, a giant six feet six inches tall and weighing two hundred and fifty pounds, when the flying whale line kinked in the boat and a man was caught and jerked overboard by the running whale and dragged with frightful speed until finally released by his limbs giving way to the strain. When rescued and brought on board, in the words of an eyewitness:

> ... it was found that a portion of the hand including four fingers had been torn away, and the foot sawed through at the ankle, leaving only the great tendon and the heel suspended to the lacerated stump. From the knee downward the muscular flesh had been rasped away by the line, leaving the protruding bone enveloped in a tangled mat of tendons and bleeding arteries. Saved from drowning, the man seemed likely to meet a more cruel death, unless some one had the nerve to perform the necessary amputation. At that time the New Bedford ships were the only ones that carried surgical instruments to meet such a case. But Captain Jim was not the man to let any one perish on slight provocation. He had his carving knife, carpenter's saw and a fish-hook. The injury was so frightful and the poor fellow's groans and cries so touching, that several of the crew fainted in their endeavors to aid the captain in the operation, and others sickened and turned away from the sight. Unaided, the captain then lashed his screaming patient to the carpenter's bench, amputated the leg and dressed the hand as best he could.

The heroism of both patient and operator was rewarded, for the man survived and ultimately reached the United States, to be for many years, as the narrator piously concludes, "another living monument of God's mercy," and he adds: "In my opinion Captain Jim suffered the most in that operation because he couldn't scream to let off his feelings."

In the earlier years even a supply of drugs was not regularly provided, but later a medicine chest with its book of directions was made part of the routine equipment, and another charge of one or two dollars was added to the already long list of items deducted from the whaleman's "lay." The medical relief afforded was not complicated by any refinements of diagnosis, for as one veteran captain says:

> Symptoms don't count in our simple practice. We open our attack with a dose of Glauber or horse salts, which takes such a strong hold on the patient that he is bound to confess we are doing something for him. It may happen that the patient grows worse, and a dose of castor oil to work off the salts is our next resource. He takes hope in the moving evidences of the medicine; and the more he endures the more he hopes. Should oil fail us, the ulterior of our modern healing art is to administer a rousing dose of calomel, with the intention that this shall work off salts, oil, and itself. In severe cases we repeat the entire course, and either kill or cure.

One medically interesting aspect of the whaleman's life that has not received the consideration it perhaps deserves is the influence such an unnatural existence may have had on the psychology of those subjected to it. The perils, the hardships, and the enforced close confinement in crowded quarters with exasperating and often quarrelsome associates during the long intervals of appalling monotony when whales were scarce must have had a deteriorating effect on morale and mental reactions, so that under such stress inferior personalities already near the border line to start with could easily give way, and possibly this explains to some extent the sadistic brutality and cruelty that were not infrequent. Captain Ahab's insane obsession in *Moby Dick* at once comes to mind, and one writer, C. B. Hawes, reproduces extracts from several whaling logs which indicate a definite strain of melancholia in the captains who wrote them. He believes that much information of interest to psychiatrists is to be found in the old manuscript records of life at sea, and expresses the conviction, reached after reading hundreds of log-books and sea journals, that the whalers had on board a disproportionate number of the mentally deranged as compared with the general run of seafaring men. It is a plausible suggestion and might repay investigation by students of abnormal psychology.

We find ourselves ending as we began, oddly enough and quite without intention, with an allusion to the lore of the psychologist. Perhaps this is as it should be, for after all no study of human endeavor can be significant without a consideration of the driving force behind it, and never has man's spirit vindicated itself more triumphantly than in the epic of his activities at sea. If the picture that has been presented of the existence of the early sailor seems unduly full of shadows, it must not be forgotten that somber colors are necessarily inherent in any depiction of medical conditions in former days, and that we have been viewing life at sea from its darkest aspect. That it had its brighter facets is undeniable; the very hardships stimulated manhood and bred a sturdy race of human beings whose courage and endurance will forever be an inspiration. From the earliest days the mariner has symbolized fortitude and daring, and even Rome's most polished poet felt this when he exclaimed, two thousand years ago: "Stout oak and triple bronze must have encased the heart of him who first entrusted his frail bark to the savage sea".

> Illi robur et aes triplex
> Circa pectus erat, qui fragilem truci
> Commisit pelago ratem
> Primus.
>
> Horace, *Odes,* III, 9.

IV

THE EVOLUTION OF THE HUMAN BRAIN

BY

FREDERICK TILNEY, M.D.

PROFESSOR OF NEUROLOGY, COLLEGE OF
PHYSICIANS AND SURGEONS, COLUMBIA UNIVERSITY

IV

THE EVOLUTION OF THE HUMAN BRAIN

THERE are two words in this title which for a long time have not enjoyed the full benefits of popular favor. One of them is "evolution" and the other is "brain." Perhaps the remaining word, "human" may supply a saving grace but, in these parlous times, even that possibility is dubious.

It is not difficult to find the reason for the standing grudge against evolution. The ape is the chief source of irritation. Surely it is far from a pleasing thought to consider him as an ancestor of our otherwise distinguished selves. There is no escaping the fact, however, that the unattractive anthropoid is the bar sinister in the evolutionary theory. He is also, to many people at least, the entire gist of this theory. That we are descended from monkeys is rather generally accepted as the true meaning of evolution. This view, at best, is a most superficial way of looking at it. No scientist to-day believes that any one of the living apes is ancestral to man. These animals belong to families totally divergent from the human family. They have ascended well up into the trees. Here, doubtless, they will remain quite as unconcerned in human origin as they are innocent of participation in it.

Whatever interest we may have in evolution should not, therefore, center in the ape-kind. The line of our ancestry reaches far back of them through millions of years. We were in the making long before there were any apes on earth. They, in their tree life, merely showed the way which shaped our course toward humanity. If we wish properly to acknowledge our hereditary indebtedness we would be forced to recognize in our family tree that highly important line of mammals which first introduced the customs of tree living. Back of them are still older lines which deserve equal ancestral credit. Here are found those animals without the existence of which we should never have arrived. Among these is that vast assortment of creatures which made their appearance in the Age of Reptiles. All of these reptilians were, in their turn, indebted for existence to earlier amphibians and fish, their progenitors during the long Age of Fish. Thus the true line of vertebrate evolution leads us from fish to man. Not until we realize the meaning of this long lineage does the vital, the inspiring significance of evolution become clear. In this way it is possible to sense the irresistible force that has carried animal life onward and upward through the ages. This force may be and probably is still at work. It may still carry us upward.

Here is a viewpoint which should make an urgent appeal for thoughtful consideration. In it are many suggestions concerning further human advancement, many possibilities for improvements and readjustments in human relations and behavior.

Further than this, it is not my intention to be an apologist either for evolution or the human brain. Both have plenty of energetic detractors; both have every assurance of a more or less permanent place wherever people permit or encourage themselves to think.

There are certain problems and questions about the brain, however, which have interested me deeply and for a long time. I trust they may interest the reader. In the first place, there is this question. What kind of a start did the brain get in life? Did it begin its career, full blown, in all its present glory and distinction? Did it ever begin at all or was it, purely and simply, a creative miracle? Was it ever something more humble and less complex than the master organ of the self-styled Homo sapiens? The answer to this last question is yes—unaccountable billions of times the answer is in the affirmative. For in every one of us, in every man, woman, and child, in every human being who ever drew breath of life, the brain has had a most simple, a most humble, a most obscure beginning. It is so simple, so humble, so obscure, that no man, however learned or sapient he may be, has ever yet been able to say just when and where and what that beginning is. The nearest we can come to it is to say that somewhere in that embryonic dawn, when a new life has touched the lowest horizons of existence, the brain begins to take shape. Watch it from then on as it slowly evolves from the indiscriminate embryonic mass and takes its appointed place. Follow its course and its changes, day by day, week by week, month by month. At length out of the indefinite matrix of daughter cells derived from a single fertilized mother cell, there is formed a complete, new human being whose life and activities are controlled by the most complex of organs, the human brain.

EMBRYONIC DEVELOPMENT

At that critical moment of emergence when the first signs of a brain can be recognized, the appearance of this future commanding organ is that of a thin plate of cells—*the neural plate stage.*

A few hours later the plate is converted into a long narrow groove bounded on either side by a rising neural fold—*the neural groove and fold stage.*

A little later the neural folds meet and fuse down the middle of the back and form a long tube, *the neural tube.*

Even while this tube is forming, one end of it begins to expand. This is the head-end and here the brain develops. The rest of the tube forms the spinal cord.

Almost from the beginning the head- or brain-end of the tube begins to specialize. By further expansions it forms a forebrain, a midbrain and a hindbrain. Each of these divisions has charge of certain definite activities of our lives.

In many ways the forebrain is the most spectacular of the brain expansions. It grows more rapidly. Out of it develop the two great hemispheres of the brain, which overshadow all other parts just as they dominate every feeling, every thought, every act of human life.

Even after these hemispheres are well defined, say around the sixth month of fetal life, they are still very primitive in their development. The billions of nerve cells in them upon which we depend for all our deliberate reactions, our thoughts, our speech, are still in the formative stages. All of these cells must yet undergo a long process of ripening and growth; (a) They must acquire fiber connections with myriads of adjacent and distant cells. (b) The fiber connections must become specially insulated to permit of the most effective intercommunication.

At the time of birth the hemispheres are richly convoluted but nonetheless thoroughly immature. They still have before them long and tedious periods of ripening, through infancy, through childhood, through adolescence. Theoretically they should attain maturity at some time early in adult life. It might easily be questioned how many human brains actually reach full maturity. Many reasons stand in the way, such as physical or social or educational or economic handicaps. Indeed it is doubtful whether the average of the human race ever develops more than a quarter of the brain's potential power.

However this may be, there can be no doubt whatsoever that, in every human being, the brain, from its extremely vague beginning, passes through a series of developmental steps by which an indefinite embryonic mass of cells becomes a highly complex adult structure capable of regulating the most complicated workings of nature, that is, the reactions of men and women.

It also seems beyond dispute that this growth of the human brain, from its inception to its completion, is, in the strictest sense and in every other sense, an evolution, an unfolding, a development, by gradual modification, from the simplest structural expression to the highest differentiation of organized matter.

RECAPITULATION

But this is not all. The human embryo does much more than tell the story of its own evolution. It repeats an even longer and greater story of the many stages through which animal life has passed to become human.

This embryonic repetition of the entire course of animal evolution has been called "recapitulation." Applied to the body as a whole, there may be serious objections to it as a principle. One thing seems certain, however; when applied to the evolution of the brain it apparently holds good every step of the way.

As in the human embryo there were at first no signs of anything that resembled a brain, so the first manifestations of animal life on this planet were devoid of any semblance of such an organ.

In fact, the first animals had no distinct organs of any kind. They lived and had their entire being in a single cell. How similar they were in this respect to the very beginning of every new human individual which also starts its career as a single cell. Many varieties of these simple animals are still living. They form a large class of organisms which are known as *Protozoa.* A good example of the protozoa is the *amœba.* Most of these minute single-celled animals are harmless. Some, however, have acquired a deservedly evil reputation among men, such for instance as the *Amœba histolytica* which causes amœbic dysentery or the *Trypanosome gambiense,* which is the cause of the African sleeping sickness or the plasmodium malaria, an almost universal enemy of mankind.

The first appearance of these tiny animals came very early in the earth's history. Later, instead of living a lonely isolated life, some of the protozoans began to collect in colonies, and, just as is the case with the single cell which starts the existence of each new human being, a community cellular life took the place of single cellular blessedness. Volvox is an excellent example of the colony-forming protozoa. Most of the colonized cells of these minute animals are on the outside, forming a hollow sphere. They are equipped with fine hairs which, by their constant motion, keep the animal rolling around in the water like a hollow rubber ball. In this manner it seeks and finds its food and thus also it may escape when threatened. But not all of the cells of Volvox are on the outside of the animal. A number of them are tucked away from the actual surface. These are the sex cells to which is entrusted the important duty of reproduction.

Even at this time in the history of the earth, although animal life had been in the process of development for millions of years, there was still no sign of anything like a brain. Forces, however, which would eventually bring such an organ into existence were already at work. Perhaps at this great distance it may be difficult to recognize their exact nature as they began to act at this particular stage of animal life. They were present, nonetheless, faintly discernible like the first streaks of dawn which precede the sunrise. This figure of speech may seem to imply that in the end, the brain was the actual sun destined to rise above the horizon of animal life and ultimately to dominate all progressive achievement. The remainder of this record must prove whether this is an extravagant figure or not.

Everything that we perceive about us in the modern world bears witness to what has been going on in the ancient world since the beginning of earthly time—an advance from the simple to the complex. A more complex type of animal organization was first seen in simplest metazoans such as the sponges (Porifera). These animals differed from the protozoans, even the colonized protozoans, because the individual cells had lost most of their separate independence. All of the cells were now incorporated as parts of a single living individual and each cell was thus definitely subordinated to the interests of the whole. The distinction between cells was still more important. The outer cells now formed a covering or skin called the *ectoderm*. The inner cells constituted the wall of a cavity which might be likened to the lining of the stomach and called the *entoderm*. Many minute openings or pores in the outer covering established communication by means of small canals with the inner cavities of the animal. Through these pores water is inhaled and carries with it particles of food which are absorbed.

It was at this critical point that a decisive factor leading to the formation of the brain made its appearance. Some of the deep cells around the pores of the sponge formed "muscles." Their obvious purpose was by contracting to regulate the flow of water through the animal's system. That function was highly important by itself. But the actual introduction of this new mechanism for producing motion was, in many ways, far more important. Here was a distinct innovation in the history of animal life—a cell or group of cells endowed with the power to contract—a new motor device which opened up untold possibilities enabling animals to move about over the earth, in the water and through the air.

Whatever great advantages there might have been in these new motor mechanisms, there also were inherent weaknesses. Motors of this kind, scattered diffusely about in the animal and left to act when and how they might be disposed, could easily defeat cooperative efforts.

Like all motors combined to serve a common purpose, they must needs be properly linked together. They needed not only a harness but a supervisor to guide them. It was probably out of this need that a nervous system and especially the brain arose.

The first step in this direction was taken when certain simple animals like sea anemones and hydras made their appearance. These animals are equipped with muscles in several parts of their bodies. Some of them have the power to move about, to crawl slowly from place to place. They are also able to move their many tentacles and thus reach out to grasp food. Each of the parts must be mutually adjusted to the others. It must act with the right rhythm, with the proper force, at the right time. Such delicate adjustment could not be left to chance; so that, in consequence of these requirements many cells were set aside and specialized as timers, signalers and despatchers. They acted more or less like independent stations, each serving separate districts, such as the individual tentacles. These independent stations ultimately earned the title of *nerve cells.* In them the first elements needed for the organization of the brain made their appearance. These nerve cells at first were scattered and had only limited communications by means of nerve fibers. In the truest sense they were the foundation stones of the brain just as the loosely arranged cells in the neural plate of the human embryo represent the essential elements of the nervous system.

The next step of progress can almost be anticipated. It consisted of consolidation, a merging of the scattered nerve cells to form a centralized system. Following this merger, the new consolidation branched out in numerous directions until a new arrangement in the muscles of the body occurred. At this juncture certain animals appeared whose bodies were elongated and slender. Their muscles were disposed in straight rows, one behind the other. Such an arrangement had definite advantages for transportation and locomotion. It was utilized by such animals as the flat worms (Platyhelminthes). Many of the nerve cells and fibers became concentrated in the head-end of these animals. This head region of the nervous system, as in the human embryo, became somewhat expanded and, in a general way, took the lead in directing the activities of locomotion. The animal now possessed a definite head which contained a brain to preside over the rest of the body.

If all this long process of successive upbuilding of the brain in animal life seems mysterious and almost miraculous, especially from its feeble beginnings in a single cell, is it actually more remarkable than the commonplace, everyday miracle that has resulted in the development and birth of all newly created animals since the dawn of time? The offspring of each species—fish or fowl, beast or man—has its beginning in a single cell. It passes through stages of cell colonization, of cellular differentiation, of specialization of cells to form organs for the various functions of life. Summarized thus briefly these successive stages necessary to bring the brain into existence may appear unimpressive. From nerve cell to brain is a few short words in print; but it required millions of years for these slowly advancing steps to attain even the humble level of the flat worms.

DEVELOPMENT OF BETTER BRAINS

With the head at length in the proper place to serve as the leader of the animal's activity, vast horizons of life still lay ahead. Better mechanisms were needed for a more successful struggle with existence.

By degrees more highly developed animals, such as bees, ants, beetles, and other insects made their appearance. Their brains were much better organized than those of the lowly worms. On the other hand, fragility of body structure and the necessity of developing an external armor imposed serious handicaps upon them. They were badly in need of an inside central axis to give them greater support and flexibility. This need foreshadowed the advent of the backboned animals. Certain invertebrates called *chordates* developed a rod-like structure which ran through the middle of their bodies and served as a central support. In some instances, this rod-like structure known as the *notochord* or *chorda dorsalis* occurs only in the anterior end of the body. Such animals form a group known as the *hemichordates* (example, Balanoglossus). In another group, the *urochordates* (Tunicates or ascidians) the chorda is restricted to the tail. Still a third group, the *cephalochordates* of which the lancelet (Amphioxus) is the outstanding example, possesses a notochord extending the entire length of the body and head.

Although all zoölogists are not in agreement as to the line of transition from the invertebrates to the backboned animals, there are certain reasons which favor the ancestral relationship just suggested. The existence of some portion of the notochord, the tubular nervous system occupying a position dorsal to the chorda and the close resemblance of the respiratory system to gill-slits afford strong indications that it was out of this chordate ancestry that the vertebrates took origin.

In any event the highest of the chordates, Amphioxus, has sufficient structural features to proclaim its close relation to backboned animals. These structural features include: (a) A longitudinal skeletal axis consisting of the notochord. (b) A dorsal nervous system. (c) A series of gill slits. (d) A musculature arrangement in a series of 60 myotomes or muscular segments symmetrically grouped about the notochord.

THE BRAIN FROM FISH TO MAMMALS

There are several other claimants to the honor of starting the highly progressive stock of vertebrates. Some authorities give the credit to lowly creatures like the starfish group (echinoderms). Others are in favor of animals not unlike the horseshoe-crab (Limulus). But the first recognizable forerunners of the progressive backboned animals were the ostracoderm fishes. They became extinct long ago and can now be identified only by their fossil remains. With the coming of the fish, the brain, already well developed in certain lower creatures, had greater opportunity to advance along more advantageous lines.

The fish, in one particular at least, showed higher

specialization. It was built for speed in locomotion. The shape of its body, the arrangement of its muscles, the position of its fins, the design of its head and the form of its tail gave it many advantages over lower animals, so much so in fact, that they became highly predatory to other forms of life. The fish also possesses powerful and remarkable eyes. It has most delicate organs for smell and an effective apparatus for taste. In fact all of the senses of the body are so thoroughly organized that each one of them has its own special department in the brain. Yet in spite of these superior arrangements there were still decided deficiencies in the central mechanism regulating the energy turnover. The fish had little or no power to withhold its reactions. Its behavior was highly impulsive. Impressions from the outside world produced almost immediate responses. Rapid reactions of this kind precluded a wide range of acts which characterize deliberate and thoughtful behavior.

The brain mechanism for the most ample kind of life was not yet present at this stage of animal development. It did begin to make its appearance when certain of the fish (Crossopterygians) assumed a partial adjustment to life on land. These adventurous pioneers managed to crawl out of the muddy waters at times when there was a lack of oxygen or when the supply of food was insufficient. They set on foot the progressive changes which gave rise to the fore and hind limbs of such amphibians as the frogs. When these latter animals had made their appearance nearly all of the fundamental problems of the vertebrate brain had been solved. Nevertheless there was still the need for certain expansion in brain power and these, in some part, were met during the next succeeding age of reptiles. The ancient handicap of almost instantaneous reaction, which imposed such serious limitations on the life of the fish, had not been entirely overcome by the amphibian or by the reptile. These animals still lacked the brain machinery needed for the deliberate and varied actions of the most effective life. They had not altogether escaped from the ancient tyrannies of automatic response and reflex reaction.

At length, the mammals, throughout the period of their long progressive age, introduced the final detail of brain perfection. The secret of this perfecting detail was the addition of a new brain mechanism never possessed by animals before this time and in fact never possessed by animals other than the mammals. Great and new areas of the cerebral hemispheres now came into existence to form the new cortex or gray matter covering each hemisphere. In this way billions of new cells were added to the brain. Their mere addition was important. Even more essential was their orderly arrangement in layers. With this new cortex there developed new and greater capacities for action together with far more effective adjustments to life.

THE BRAIN OF LOWER MAMMALS

When the mammals became possessed of this priceless brain equipment, the new cortex, they at once began to turn it to their own immediate advantage. It may be more strictly correct to say that this new cortex opened up avenues of opportunity which the mammals were quick to follow. At any rate, they became, from the beginning of the Age of Mammals, great adventurers and great specialists.

One of their chief specialties is the care of their young. Of course, they are not unique in this specialty because birds and even some reptiles and certain fish develop most striking nursery habits. But, all in all, the mammal is particularly well fitted for the business of parenthood. The marsupial opossum, for example, has had at least eighty-five million years' experience as a parent and is still doing an excellent job. This small mammal is called a living fossil because its skeletal structure has remained practically unchanged since the time when it was one of the contemporaries of the dinosaurs in North America. It carries and nurses its young in a pouch from the time they are ten millimeters long until they are able to forage and care for themselves. As parenthood goes, this is not a task to be lightly esteemed, for the mother has ten to thirteen young ones at a time.

What adventurers the mammals have been and how they have specialized is shown by the fact that they have occupied every one of the twelve habitat zones on earth. Professor Osborn has defined this adventuresomeness as *adaptive radiation*. Whales and porpoises have invaded the sea and make it their dwelling place. Seals and their kind live partially on land and partially in the water. Hoofed animals inhabit the plains. Bats and flying squirrels find conveyance through the air. Moles and burrowing animals live underground. The meat-eaters scent out every corner of the earth and carry on their hunting expeditions under the guidance of a wily brain.

Concerning the increased capacity of the mammals as a class, there seems to be no doubt. When we compare the actions and capabilities of such mammals as dogs, horses, elephants, or any one of the cat family, with those of the bird, or the snake, or the fish, the vast differences speak for themselves. The dog for example has, by comparison with lower vertebrates, a greatly increased capacity for getting on in life. He is capable of adapting himself to many complications incident to his associations with man. He has a much more ample repertoire of performances. He is capable of learning many intricate accomplishments. In general such learning is also true of most of the higher mammals. It is particularly true of those having a highly developed neocortex. Even aquatic mammals like seals show a remarkable degree of adaptability. They are among the most interesting of trained performers. A casual glance is sufficient to show what an excellent convoluted cortex they possess. In spite of their huge proportions and awkwardness, elephants are capable of remarkable adjustments. Their cortex is also highly developed.

Yet, however decisive the mammalian superiority in brain power may be in comparison with lower vertebrates, most mammals are held down by handicaps, restrictions, and limitations of their own. They may be perfectly well adapted for life in the water, in the air, on the plains, underground, or in the forest, but their own specializations hold them to specifically restricted adjustments. They may be well able to do the things which hoof and paw, wing and flipper, trunk and head make possible. But here their opportunities for achievement cease. In this way the progress of most mammals is held in check by numerous obstacles.

One group and one group alone escaped these serious embarrassments. They enjoyed a structural plasticity which opened for them a long road of progressive development. They began to follow a new line of progress which finally called upon the brain for its supreme development. This group of animals took its initial and main advantage from the fact that it assumed a life in the trees. Tree-living of this kind according to Professor Gregory began with late Paleocene representatives of the tree-shrew, while perfected arboreal primates first appeared in the lower Eocene. Notharctus was such a primitive, tree-living, primate. Its hands and feet were of the grasping type similar to more recent primates like lemurs and monkeys. There can be no doubt that ancestral primates had, at this early date, learned to make their ways with security through the leafy highways of the trees.

DAWN AND DEVELOPMENT OF THE PRIMATE BRAIN

We are now approaching a critical period in the history of the brain. It contains many incidents of utmost importance. Particularly noteworthy are the episodes which favored the production of humanoid traits in the animal kingdom. These traits showed many manlike tendencies which much later were to appear full-fledged in the human race. They were from the first limited to a single, highly interesting order of mammals. This fact seems somewhat strange, because from the beginning of the Age of Mammals sixty-five million years ago, a great variety of new animals came into existence. That a single order, out of all this vast number, was selected to develop human resemblances must hold the secret of some potent influence. Such an influence was definitely at work. Little by little it changed and reshaped the structure of the body until at length there appeared a race of animals so human in their organization that they might well have been the forerunners of mankind.

It would not be easy to conceive the kind of modifications in structure which could produce the form of man from a whale, a horse, or a dog. Such animals have many specializations of their own which would require extensive simplification before any satisfactory attempt at remodeling could be undertaken. This is not true of the monkey-kind. In many of their essential features these animals resemble men and that is why they are placed under the name of *primates* in the same bracket with man. Their arrival on the scene marked the beginning of a new and epoch-making day in the animal kingdom. We shall be interested to follow the advances that occurred in their mental capacities as they slowly made their progressive strides forward. We shall be particularly struck by those changes showing the chief lines of progress which the human brain must have followed.

Passing upward from the lowest of the primates into the higher families of the apes, we shall not only observe a pronounced increase in manlike tendencies, but as the great anthropoids at length become human in miniature and then almost human, we shall recognize a brain which more and more resembles the brain of man.

As in other spheres of life, there are class distinctions among the primates. The lowest of the monkey-kind include the lemurs, tarsiers and all of the New World monkeys. In the next higher stratum are monkeys of the Old World. The anthropoid apes occupy the top rank and include the gibbon, orang-utan, chimpanzee, and gorilla. They are nearest to man both in appearance and in habits.

BEHAVIOR AND BRAIN OF THE LOWEST MONKEYS

The lowest monkeys show but little advance over lower mammals. Whatever progressive advantages they possess should be attributed to new facilities in adjustment to tree-living and also to the development of grasping hands and feet.

Their mentality is essentially primitive. Professor Thorndyke has made most careful studies of the behavior of several different species of South American monkeys. He believes that they represent a certain advance from the more generalized mammal toward man. All of this is an advance due to the brain acting with increased delicacy.

In following the actual brain development through the primates to man, it has been necessary to select a few outstanding cerebral features, several of which can be subjected to measurement. These features include the Central, Sylvian, and Simian fissures, the Parietal Lobe for body sense, the Temporal Lobe for hearing, the Occipital Lobe for vision, and the Frontal Lobe for the higher faculties. Two highly important structures on the base are also included, that is, the pons Varolii or bridge, held by some authorities as an index of intelligence and the pyramid which indicates the degree of the neocortical control over all voluntary action.

The fissures and lobes of the lower monkeys show some improvements over the general mammalian pattern—enough at least to justify the assumption that we are now dealing with a higher order of brain organization. The pontile index shows definite advances from lemur which is .055, tarsiers .057, marmoset .095 to the South American howling monkey which is .103. The pyramidal index for these four primates is respectively .110, .032, .064 and .137.

In this manner the first primate steps toward a more efficient type of brain were taken. It seems clear that the conditions of tree-life incited and successfully urged them forward.

BRAIN AND BEHAVIOR OF THE INTERMEDIATE MONKEYS

A good example of these monkeys is the *Macacus* or Indian monkey. Mr. Kipling described them in his famous "Road Song of the Bandar-Log,"

> Jabber it quickly and all together
> Excellent! Wonderful! Once again!
> Now we are talking just like men
> Let us pretend we are—never mind
> Brother, thy tail hangs down behind.

These monkeys are constantly in motion when awake. Always amusing, the macaque is sure to hold the attention of any human audience. He lives in a busy world of jabbering mischievous animals continuously up to something but seldom getting anything done except, perhaps, to fill his cheek pouches as full as he can.

Dr. Kinnaman, who has made studies on the mentality of these monkeys, believes that they have attained a higher level of intelligence than the New World monkeys. Professor Thorndyke and Dr. Hobhouse are of the opinion that macaques have limited powers of reasoning. Professor Yerkes, after a longer and more systematic study with experimental methods better suited to the problem, agrees with Professor Thorndyke that the macaques may have a certain number of limited ideas.

The brain of *Macacus* shows definite advances when compared with that of the lower monkeys. Not only are the fissures deeper and better defined but the several lobes are larger and more extensively convoluted. The pontile index is .150 and pyramidal coefficient .147.

BRAIN AND BEHAVIOR OF GIBBON AND ORANG-UTAN

Manlike tendencies are more pronounced in the smaller anthropoid apes. Certain traits of this kind are obvious in the gibbon which is able to stand up, walk and run upon two legs. This he does a little awkwardly but not unlike a human being. The locomotion of these animals in the trees is totally different from that of other monkeys. Gibbons employ their arms almost exclusively, swinging from branch to branch, with the legs tucked up close to the body. This is an important and provocative change in the arboreal methods of transportation. In the first place, swinging from one limb to another elongated the forearm and fingers. The second effect produced by this kind of locomotion, which is called *branchiation,* was the progressive drawing of the body more and more into the erect posture.

If the gibbon's resemblances to man are somewhat vague, it is possible to recognize certain tendencies which point in the human direction. His ability to assume the erect posture, to stand and run on his hind legs, his well-developed grasping hands and the marvelous coördination of his upper extremities, as displayed in his swinging gait among the branches, are all features which appear more highly developed in man.

Another, even more manlike ape is the orang-utan. He is wild and shy but possesses enormous strength which makes him more than a match for the most able-bodied man. When full grown he stands a little more than four feet in height. His arms are long and slender, reaching almost to the ankles when he stands erect. The legs are relatively short. His powerful arms with their long grasping hands enable him to climb easily to the topmost branches, although he prefers to sleep low down in the tree, not over twenty or thirty feet from the ground.

Professor Yerkes has contributed important studies of intelligence tests applied to the orang. These tests were devised on what is known as the "multiple choice basis" and used with the partly grown orang, "Julius." This anthropoid persistently endeavored to gain some insight into every test situation. Although slow, he showed that the brain had at length attained the development necessary for the production of real ideas.

In the gibbon and more particularly in the orang the parietal, temporal, and occipital lobes have increased in prominence. At this stage it is possible to speak of a well-developed frontal lobe. The gradual emergence of this lobe is one of the features in the anthropoid which leads up to the outstanding characteristic of the human brain.

The pontile index in the gibbon is .200; in the orang it is .300. The pyramidal coefficient of the gibbon is .138, of the orang .160.

BRAIN AND BEHAVIOR OF THE CHIMPANZEE

The chimpanzee has established a reputation for many valuable qualities. He is a performer of no mean talents and often as a comedian earns a large salary. He is likewise famous as an acrobat.

One of the best studies of the chimpanzee comes to us as an echo of the World War. Some years ago the Prussian Academy of Science established at Teneriffe in the Canary Islands a special station equipped for the study of the great manlike apes. It was here that Professor Köhler found himself during the war and here he remained interned with nine chimpanzees for two years. During this time he lived with these animals largely shut off from the rest of the world by the naval blockade. The results of his experience and studies are given in a remarkable narrative published both in English and German called the *Mentality of Apes*. In this work his chief purpose was to test the intelligence of the larger anthropoids by especially improvised methods.

He found that the champanzees were able to learn the use of certain simple implements like straws and twigs in lieu of spoons. In many respects, such as in play or hunting, the animals had numerous human resemblances. Several of them developed fine and somewhat dangerous marksmanship in throwing sticks and stones. Being of a buoyant and mirthful nature, the apes derived evident pleasure from clowning and masquerade. Perhaps their most constructive abilities were shown in their manufactures and buildings. They were able to construct useful instruments to help them in obtaining food. There can be no doubt that the chimpanzee, in a modest way, does manufacture implements which help him to gain his ends.

All of these animals ultimately developed some degree of constructive engineering ability. This ability grew out of their learning to pile boxes in order to reach objects suspended over their heads. After they had built a tower-like structure of this kind the long bamboo rod came in handy as a means of bringing the suspended banana to the ground.

The chimpanzee has certain definitely surgical interests. This applies especially to the removal of splinters from the hands and feet of his companions. Professor Köhler himself, having once suffered from such an accident, ventured to allow one of the chimpanzees to perform the necessary operation. The clinical procedure was skilfully and successfully accomplished.

Almost all observers credit the chimpanzee with unusual good fellowship. In the army encampments in Africa they are the much-prized pets of the officers. At mess dinners the chimpanzee often manifests a keen liking for good wines. Like his human companions, he sometimes rises to hilarious heights.

Should doubts remain concerning the superior, almost human capacities of the chimpanzee, these may be soon put at rest by inspection of his brain. This organ is human in miniature. It reveals the neocortical means by which this animal has acquired his new and extensive powers of learning, his greater understanding, his better capacity for adjustment.

All of the cerebral fissures have a close resemblance to the fissures of the human brain. The lobes are highly convoluted and follow a pattern in all respects similar to that of man except that the convolutions in the chimpanzee are less complex. The frontal lobe in the chimpanzee is more extensive than in the orang, or any other of the lower primates. The counterpart of almost every human convolution is present in somewhat simplified form. The pontile index has a value of .400 while the pyramidal coefficient, indicating the degree of neocortical control over skilled acts, is .172.

THE BRAIN AND BEHAVIOR OF THE GORILLA

The largest member of the ape world is the gorilla. There is some dispute to-day as to the place he occupies among the primates and also as to what rating his intelligence deserves. Neither of these questions can be settled at present.

For many centuries, the gorilla has had an unsavory reputation because of his savage disposition. The celebrated explorer, Carl Akeley, felt that this huge and ungainly animal had been done a real injustice in this respect. Instead of being an incorrigible brute he is in reality timid and retiring. It was due to Mr. Akeley's efforts that the king of Belgium set aside a large territory in the Belgian Congo as a gorilla sanctuary. Here, in the vicinity of three extinct volcanoes, Mt. Keno, Mt. Karissimbi and Mt. Visake, Mr. Akeley hoped that a biological station might be established for the further study of the gorilla's behavior.

Some young gorillas have already been subjected to prolonged observation. Miss Alyse Cunningham found John Daniel the First in a show window as an advertisement for a well-known shop in London. The little animal was suffering from influenza and rickets. Miss Cunningham took this infant gorilla into her home and nursed him through his sickness. In the next three years he reached the weight of 112 pounds and attained the height of 3 feet, 4½ inches. Meanwhile he acquired many of the adjustments necessary to fit him as an interesting if wholly unusual member of the household.

We are indebted to Miss Cunningham for an excellent account of his life which indicates the extent to which this great ape may be trained and educated. Little John, immediately after his recovery from influenza, began to show some singularly childlike emotions. He was gentle and affectionate in response to the tender care he received. If he were left to himself at night he would shriek from fear and loneliness. Perhaps he remembered the long and cheerless nights when he was a Christmas exhibit in the department store. In any event it was necessary for Miss Cunningham to coax, soothe and pet him until she allayed his fears. At length he would become quiet and fall asleep.

At the end of six weeks he was thoroughly housebroken. He was then allowed the freedom of the house. He showed strong likes and dislikes in the matter of food. There was one feature in this respect that always puzzled Miss Cunningham. Generally speaking John was not a thief. He manifested average honesty, but when it came to food, he much preferred to steal it than have it given to him. It was difficult to understand the motive underlying this course of action. Some facts seemed to indicate a real satisfaction in stealing due to an outcropping of deep, inherent tendencies. Perhaps it was the working out of that ancient predatory drive to go and get what was wanted without leave or invitation which later was to become such a devastating urge in prehistoric, primitive and modern man.

While he was growing up, he was always fond of people and liked to have them visit him in his home. On such occasions he was given to showing off like a child. He always took afternoon tea with the family and also liked his demi-tasse of coffee after dinner. The family estimate of him was generally high. Incidentally, John Daniel had a very good opinion of himself. He was quite well poised and self-contained. Nothing seemed to ruffle him. He seemed to believe that his own estimate of himself was shared by others and appeared confident that every one was delighted to see him. Often he would stand on the window-sill and throw up the shade. In a short time a crowd would collect in the street to watch this unusual sight. He enjoyed such publicity immensely. Once in a while, if the crowd grew very large, he would deliberately pull down the shade in their faces and run away shrieking with laughter in a way that seemed to indicate that he was conscious of having perpetrated a huge joke on his audience outside. Of course, this entire reaction and the motives underlying it are open to several interpretations. Skeptics will say that the version here given endows the gorilla with attributes more human than he could possibly possess. However that may be, those who actually observed these performances were impressed by the fact that John Daniel did act in a seemingly human manner.

As the years passed he became more devotedly attached to the family. When he was six years old, through a misunderstanding which his owners always regretted, John was sold to a circus. He was taken across the Atlantic to New York. Here, after a month's separation from his devoted friends, during which time he refused to take food and showed every sign of real homesickness, he died in the tower of the old Madison Square Garden in April, 1921.

As an interesting sequel to this history, Miss Cunningham secured another gorilla which she called John Daniel the Second. These two great apes resembled each other closely in their emotional reactions and in their responses to training. John the Second was perhaps a less likable individual and had a disposition more in keeping with the ancient repute of gorillas. Several years ago, while he was visiting New York, a number of scientists were invited to have tea with him at a certain fashionable hotel. On this occasion, the troglodyte host was found seated in a comfortable chair. He displayed much gravity and apparent enjoyment as he drank from a cup of tea. During the course of conversation John was not, for an instant, the actual center of attention. Suddenly he dashed across the room with unbelievable swiftness and attacked one of his professorial visitors with repeated blows of both fists in the neighborhood of the solar plexus. With equal swiftness he hopped over the foot of the bed and from this point of vantage watched the discomfiture of his guest.

Mr. Akeley's attractive prospect of a biological station in the African Congo for the study of the gorilla is inspiring. It will, however, require more than inspiration to induce a number of professors of my acquaintance to enter the African jungle with the purpose of studying the allegedly docile and otherwise pleasantly coöperative gorilla.

Other young animals of this species have been studied in captivity. One of them, Congo the Second, has been the basis of the most careful and scientific study thus far made. In a book called *The Mind of a Gorilla,* Professor Yerkes has given us another of his brilliant works on animal behavior. All of his observations are illuminating and helpful in understanding the brain of this great troglodyte.

The gorilla's brain is larger and weighs more than that of any other anthropoid ape. In many other respects it is nearest to the brain of man. The central fissure forms the boundary of a well-defined, highly developed frontal lobe. All of the other fissures and lobes are more prominent and complexly convoluted. Indicative of his powers to adjust himself to a strenuous life, the gorilla's pontile index gives him a rating of .480 which is still higher than in the case of the agile chimpanzee. Most interesting in this connection is the fact that the pyramidal coefficient in the gorilla is .161 which is considerably less than in the chimpanzee. The pyramid, it will be recalled, indicates the degree of skill that an animal has in controlling its voluntary movements, that is, in making its muscles act in many and varied ways according to the dictates of the will. That the agile, acrobatic chimpanzee should surpass the clumsier, slower moving gorilla in this particular might be expected. If any final estimation is justified at the present time, the gorilla's brain appears to be the most advanced of the apes and is, in fact, almost human.

THE ARRIVAL OF MAN

The brain had passed through certain preliminary stages long before man made his appearance on the scene. Its basic patterns had been perfected. Its most important mechanisms had been improved. In those preparatory days, all manner of animals inhabited the earth—fish, amphibians, reptiles, birds, and mammals. They were the stepping stones of progress. When at length the first members of our family arrived, their brains were barely human and they themselves were most crude human beings. There was a certain triumph in their advent, however, for at last there were men. They were to inaugurate a new age which was to be called the Age of Man, and was to differ from all preceding ages by the steadily increasing products of human achievement. But the brain of these men was relatively small in its capacity and still unrefined in many of its structural details. Hundreds of thousands of years were necessary for such a brain as this to attain its highest efficiency. To most of us who are accustomed to reckon time as the hours between breakfast and dinner or at most as the proverbial three score years and ten, these long periods sound fabulous and fantastic. In contemplating the past our vision usually stops short at the beginning of history, five to six thousand years ago. Such a focus is unfortunately near-sighted. It leaves us insensitive to the much longer prehistoric period. Yet through all this unrecorded time, man struggled upward to achieve those successes which at length established the Age of the Frontal Lobe. Much evidence of this vast prehistoric period is now available. It tells us of at least four extinct races of man. Carefully examined, it reveals what the early members of our family must have been when the long human journey first started.

In all his races, living and extinct, man constitutes the sixth family in the primate suborder, *Anthropoidea* (manlike). This family is known as the *Hommidæ* (men of all types). The progenitors of the human family split off from a common primate stock at some time early in the Oligocene. At this critical juncture, probably twenty-five million years ago, two great branches of the suborder parted company. Thenceforth they developed independently of each other. The first branch from this common stem gave rise to human races. From the second branch arose the great modern anthropoid apes including the orang-utan, the chimpanzee and the gorilla.

The question often arises—How is the antiquity of human remains determined? The principal criteria are four in number. First, the age in geologic time of the stratum within which the remains are found. Second, the fossil remains of other animals associated with the fossil remains of man, whether these be of still living forms or entirely extinct species. Third, the human artifacts, that is, implements, weapons, ornaments, and other objects produced by human hands. Fourth, the structural characteristics as to teeth, skull, and other parts of the skeleton which distinguish these fossil people from living races.

THE JAVAN APE-MAN: PITHECANTHROPUS ERECTUS

Probably the oldest, most primitive of extinct races is the Ape-man of Java who, although definitely human, had many simian qualities. He possessed a head and face not unlike those of an ape but his brain was nearly twice the size of any simian (940 c.c.). It was this advantage which assured him an unassailable place as a member of the human family. The fossil remains of the Ape-man were discovered in 1891 by a Dutch army surgeon, Dr. Eugen DuBois. He made the discovery on the Bengawan River in Central Java, finding almost the entire skullcap of this primitive man. It is estimated that Pithecanthropus lived somewhere between five hundred thousand and a million years ago.

The striking feature about the brain of the ape-man is the great expansion which has taken place in the frontal lobe. Of even greater significance are the indications of a convolution in the lower portion of the frontal lobe on the left side. In all living men this convolution is associated with the control of spoken language. It seems probable therefore that the ape-man had acquired the powers of speech. This acquisition had a decisive bearing on the destiny of humanity.

If it were possible to catalogue the chief developmental changes which determined human emergence from lower levels of animal life they doubtless would appear in the following order:

1. The development of the human foot upon which to establish the erect posture.

2. The freeing of the hand in consequence of the erect posture for the purposes of human success.

3. The expansion of sight and hearing for better appreciation of the world and the more effective guidance of action.

4. The development of speech.

5. The establishment of human personality and the development of higher mental faculties.

All of these changes were directly dependent upon the growth and higher specialization of the neocortex, particularly in the region of the frontal lobe. Most of these modifications were, to some degree, operative in the Ape-man of Java.

THE DAWN-MAN OF PILTDOWN, ENGLAND: EOANTHROPUS DAWSONI

From certain flints, with many features indicating their use as instruments, it is held probable that there were primitive men living in England at a time earlier than that assigned to the Ape-man of Java. Disputes about those early prehistoric Englishmen arise from the fact that no actual human remains of them have yet been found. This, fortunately, is not the case with the famous English Dawn-Man. This human fossil was found by Charles Dawson at Piltdown, a town in the weald of Sussex not many miles from the English Channel. The fossilized remnants consisted of a number of fragments of this extinct man's skull. In December 1912, Sir A. Smith-Woodward and Mr. Dawson presented to the Geological Society of London a reconstruction of the Piltdown skull. The announcement of this remarkable discovery made a deep stir in scientific circles. An unknown phase of early human existence was about to be revealed. The reconstructed skull impressed all who saw it as a strange blend of ape and man. Some suggested that it was the missing link for which the early followers of Darwin had earnestly sought. But whether this was the missing link or not, the Piltdown strata in Sussex told of a race of human beings who inhabited England long before history had made its feeblest beginnings. Dr. Smith-Woodward believes the fossil dated back to the early part of the Pleistocene period. Sir Arthur Keith and Professor Osborn give it far greater antiquity and assign it to some part of the Pliocene. Whatever the exact prehistoric time of the Piltdown fossil may be, it is clear that a very primitive race of men lived in England thousands of years before Cæsar's invasions, in fact ages before the ancient Celts or Goedælic Britons occupied the land. The Piltdown man is regarded by some as the direct ancestor of modern races; by others he is held to be an independent branch of the human family of quite unknown affiliations.

Several different brain-casts have been made from the reconstructed skull of the Dawn-man of England. Such differences as exist in them do not contradict the fact that this brain was undeniably human and superior to that of the Ape-man of Java.

NEANDERTHAL MAN: HOMO PRIMOGENIUS

Man's first great epoch came in the Old Stone Age (Paleolithic, which began nine hundred thousand years ago). A new and sturdy race of men gained the upper hand in Europe. This race is known as the Neanderthals. The ancestry of these remarkable people is traced back to the Heidelberg man (Paleoanthropus) who appeared about eight hundred thousand years ago and is considered the first man of the Old Stone Age. The Neanderthals have a probable antiquity of six hundred thousand years. They were hunters and the first cave-dwellers. As flint workers they made and improved many implements. Their long period of human supremacy is characterized by definite culture periods, such as the Chellean, Acheulean, and Mousterian periods.

The scattered fossils of this famous race which have been found in many different parts of Europe all tell the story of an unusually powerful people. Their arms were long and muscular, their necks thick, their legs short and slightly bent at the knees. The Neanderthal had a low retreating forehead with heavy ridges of bone arching above the eyes. The jaws were heavy, the nose broad and flat, the chin receding. All of these features must have given the Neanderthal man a brutish appearance. His brain, however, attests that far from being a lowly apelike creature, he had many of the higher human attributes.

The earliest discovery of these ancient people was made in 1848 when Lieutenant Flint found a Neanderthal skull in an old quarry at Gibraltar. These aggressive and productive people dominated Europe until well on toward the end of the Old Stone Age. The problem of their disappearance before the advances of a superior people has not yet been solved. The real secret in the failure of the old Neanderthal race and the success of the newcomers is doubtless to be found in the brain. It was the increased brain power of the Cromagnons which produced the supremacy of this last great race in the Old Stone Age. It was this power which gave Europe its first pioneers in art and which, for all mankind, opened the doors of creative imagination and appreciation of beauty in the world.

CROMAGNON MAN: HOMO SAPIENS

The Cromagnon has a probable antiquity of fifty thousand years. He has a well-developed brain and frontal lobe of thoroughly modern type. He was an effective warrior and huntsman but above all he was an artist. He employed and greatly refined the flint implements of the Old Stone Age and passed through successive cultural periods known as the Aurignacian,

Solutrean, Magdalenian and Azilian. His chief contribution to human progress was the introduction and founding of art. He was the world's first great artist.

The fate of the Cromagnon race was no exception to what had gone before or what would follow many times thereafter. Race after race, nation after nation rose and became master, declined and passed into final extinction. As the day of Cromagnon ascendancy waned a new race invaded Europe. The Old Stone Age came to its end approximately ten thousand years ago with the advent of the more vigorous Neolithic man. With the introduction of agriculture, the domestication of animals and the establishment of permanent abode, men of the New Stone Age contributed many of the essentials of modern life. The essentials included new ways of defending their claims and asserting their rights. This new assertiveness quickly led to the more sanguinary ages of Bronze and Iron with their communal equipments for offense and defense. Its influences finally spread into historic times. Ultimately these more aggressive tendencies created all of the armed camps which we are pleased to call civilization, ancient, medieval, and modern. At the end of the New Stone Age all of the direct ancestors of modern European races were established in Europe.

The dawn of history was followed by a procession of great events which began in the early Egyptian dynasties. The development of Pharaonic culture, the regal splendors of Babylonia and Chaldea, the incomparable achievements of Greece and Rome followed in rapid succession. Each of these civilizations contributed to the development of the race. Then came the eclipse of the Dark Ages in medieval times and at length the bright light of the Renaissance, the illuminating influences of which have been carried forward in the accomplishments characteristic of modern times.

This is an inspiring picture of almost uninterrupted human progress. How readily it has been taken at its face value by the most gullible of living animals, Homo sapiens. Man has been too deeply engrossed in his ancient glories and modern proficiencies to take a good look at himself. No longer than a quarter of a century ago there were reasons for the Caucasian's pride and self-assurance. Peace existed between the nations. Success filled every walk of life. Social order rested upon firm moral foundations. This was a human establishment upon which to rely. But ultimately this record of the white man brings us to a fateful midsummer afternoon in August 1914. The race has been the victim of many such self-inflicted catastrophies. Thus far it has always managed to come back and go forward again. Where it has stood still, where it has, perhaps, even fallen behind, is in the manifest lack of control over human nature.

Since his early beginnings man has grown in humanity as his brain expanded. Such a conclusion seems irresistible. Placed side by side the brain casts of the Ape-man of Java, the Dawn-man of Piltdown, the Rhodesian, the Neanderthal, the Predmast and the modern demonstrate this expansion. The brain area in which the greatest development has occurred is the frontal lobe. Its growth conveys an accurate impression of the manner in which the brain has responded to the demands made upon it. Those demands continue to be made. This fact seems to point in a hopeful direction. The human cerebrum may still be considered to be in its early youth. By most of us it is regarded as a finished product. Its long prehistoric record as we know it to-day does not support this point of view. On the contrary it makes it appear far more likely that the brain of modern man is only some intermediate stage in the ultimate development of the master organ of life.

V

THE HISTORY OF MEDICAL HISTORY

BY

HENRY E. SIGERIST, M.D.

PROFESSOR OF THE HISTORY OF MEDICINE, THE JOHNS HOPKINS UNIVERSITY

V

THE HISTORY OF MEDICAL HISTORY

MEDICAL history [1] is a relatively young field of research; for the good reason that until about a century ago ancient medicine was still alive. Medical men were familiar with the history of their craft and their books were full of historical consideration. Ancient books were studied not as historical documents but as authorities or at least as sources of information. Haller's monumental *Elementa Physiologiæ* published from 1757 to 1766 discussed not only contemporary views but physiological theories from Hippocrates on.

[1] I have discussed principles of medical history several times: first in an inaugural address at the University of Zurich, "Aufgaben und Ziele der Medizingeschichte," *Schweizerische Medizinische Wochenschrift,* Vol. 3, 1922, pp. 318-322; in an inaugural address at the University of Leipzig, "Die Geschichte der Medizin im Rahmen der Universitas Litterarum," *Deutsche Medizinische Wochenschrift,* Vol. 53, 1927, pp. 777-779, 864, 949-950; and in a paper read before the Eighth International Congress of Medical History, in Rome, in 1930, "Probleme der medizinische Historiographie," *Archiv für Geschichte der Medizin,* Vol. 24, 1931, pp. 1-18. In an Open Letter to George Sarton I tried to show that the history of medicine is not a mere chapter of the history of science but has intrinsic problems of its own (*Bulletin of the Institute of the History of Medicine, The Johns Hopkins University,* Vol. IV, 1936, pp. 1-13). If I am discussing these problems here once more, whereby I naturally must repeat some statements made in previous papers, I am doing it because my views have evolved and because these questions are particularly acute to me to-day at a time when I am working on a four-volume History of Medicine.

This attitude toward the medical past changed radically in the second half of the nineteenth century when a new medical science developed. To the average physician of that period the history of medicine appeared as the history of medical errors. Ancient medical texts were still studied but not in order to learn from them. They were investigated as sources of history. When Emile Littré in 1839 published the first volume of his edition and translation of Hippocrates he still had the general practitioner as reader in mind. When Charles Daremberg, twelve years later, began the publication of a collection of Greek medical writers he undertook it for students of history. In the beginning of our century national societies were founded for the study of medical history, and in 1905 Karl Sudhoff organized the first research institute in the field, at the University of Leipzig.

There was medical historiography before our time. Ancient and medieval writers often speculated about the origins and early beginnings of the healing art. The medical views of the various schools were listed. In the Renaissance when people were particularly interested in individual achievements, biographies of prominent physicians and bibliographies of their works were written. The bio-bibliographical approach to medical history has remained extremely popular. At the end of the seventeenth and in the beginning of the eighteenth centuries a Frenchman, Daniel le Clerc, an Englishman, J. Freind, and a German, J. H. Schulze, each wrote a history of medicine. Their books had a profound influence on medical historiography and together with Kurt Sprengel's great *Versuch einer pragmatischen Geschichte der Arzneykunde* (1821 to 1840) they established a definite pattern that has been followed more or less by every historian of medicine until to-day. They pictured the history of medicine as the history of great doctors, and their discoveries and achievements as the history of medical institutions and as the history of medical theories and ideas. Every new textbook added new materials but the basic pattern remained very much the same.

It seems to me that the time has come to break this pattern and to approach the history of medicine from a different and broader angle. Before we can do this, however, we must know what the nature and function of medical history are, in what ways the subject can and must be approached, what problems it raises and what methods of investigation it requires.

What is medical history? It, obviously, is first of all *history*. It is an historical discipline like the history of philosophy or the history of art. It, therefore, has the general historical research methods in common with all other historical disciplines. The historian proceeds analytically by investigating sources in order to be able to reconstruct the past. What is an historical source?

If on a walk we find a stone, this may be an object of scientific research to the mineralogist or geologist but is of no interest to the historian. As soon, however, as we find the slightest trace of human influence on such a stone, be it a drawing, or a sculpture, or just a few letters, the stone immediately assumes a different character. It becomes an historical document. Our first task in investigating such a document is to describe it as accurately as possible. We proceed exactly as the scientist would. Our second task, however, is strictly historical and consists in dating the document. It has to be located in time and space for it obviously makes a great difference whether such a stone is Babylonian or Greek, and whether it is fifth or third century Greek. Chronology is the iron foundation of all historical work. It is somewhat out of fashion because the time is not so far back when historians were nothing but chroniclers and it certainly is more interesting to interpret historical events than to list them. But every interpretation presupposes accurate dating of sources.

Our third task is to find out what the meaning of the document is. In the case of the stone we want to know what the signs that we found on it mean, whether they are a record or a religious symbol, or a text. We are two men facing each other: the man who centuries before created the document and I, the historian, endeavoring to understand what he meant.

In most cases the situation is still more complicated because we do not see the object of our studies; we read about it. We read about the influence of Vesalius's work. We read about the Hippocratic treatment of pneumonia. We see the facts and events in the mirror of literature—a mirror that is never quite accurate.

What are the sources of medical history? It is obvious that every object and every document can be of interest to the medical historian. Whatever men do becomes history the minute it is done. And whatever record of our activities we leave becomes an historical source. Every document that concerns the people's health is a source of medical history. Such documents are not only medical books, pictures, and objects, but endless other non-medical records as well. We must keep in mind, moreover, that the health problems of a given society are merely one aspect of a very complex set of other problems, and that the medical science of a definite period again is only one expression of the general philosophy and scientific views of the time. If we want to understand these problems we must consult an infinity of other, non-medical sources.

It is obviously impossible to investigate all sources available. If a historian intending to write a history of the World War would attempt to examine all existing documents on the subject, it would keep him busy for probably more than a century and at the end he would be so confused that he could not possibly write his book. We have to make a selection of sources, concentrating our attention on some of them and discarding others as unimportant. The scientist will find that this is an unscientific procedure; that we are introducing an arbitrary element into our investigation. This may be true, but the scientist is proceeding in a very similar way. He, too, selects his problem. When he experiments he asks nature questions. In animal experiments he creates artificial conditions and observes how the organism reacts to them.

There is an arbitrary element in every human investigation whether scientific or historical.

How do we select our sources? Which are important and which not? It all depends on the problem. If we look at a group of medical men—for example the faculty of a medical school—we will find that all individuals are different from each other. They all lead their own life, work in their laboratories and clinics on their individual problems. And yet different as they all may be, they still have a great deal in common due to the fact that they are contemporaries, living in the same country, under the same economic system. They all went through the same type of schools, studied the same classics, had experiences in common. And they all think in definite terms. The number of concepts to operate with, available at a given time, is limited, and these concepts are different to-day than they were in the Middle Ages, or in Antiquity, or in China. We cannot escape the fact that we are living in a definite period as members of a given society. If one of us thinks in entirely different terms he will not be understood, will soon find himself isolated, or may even be recognized as mentally sick.

What all these men have in common constitutes a trend which is going to stand out in history when most individual contributions will have been forgotten. We are primarily interested in these trends and the more we study them, the more we recognize that the individuals are the mere exponents of such movements, the instruments of powerful social forces.

There is another point that has to be taken into consideration, namely that the history of medicine is the history of a *techne,* of a craft. While most historical disciplines study events that happened once or creations that are unique, medical history examines skills, technics, practical achievements. We are interested in what has been done in various periods of history in order to restore and preserve health. We investigate the Hippocratic writings not only as literary documents, and not only as intellectual manifestations of fifth-century Greece. We study them because we want to know how the Hippocratic doctors treated definite diseases. And we are anxious to know, moreover, whether they did a good job or not. In other words: there will always be valuations in medical history.

It seems to me that medical history has three major fields of research. The first set of problems that we have to attack concerns the *history of disease.* We cannot understand a physician's behavior nor can we judge how he fulfilled his task unless we know what diseases he was called to fight.

Paleopathology has demonstrated that disease is as old as life itself, that it occurred long before the advent of man. The examination of fossil bones has further shown that disease manifested itself at all times in the same basic forms that we observe to-day. This was to be expected because the animal organism has a limited number of mechanisms available with which to react against lesions and these mechanisms were apparently always the same.

The incidence of disease, however, and the character of the individual diseases were very different in various periods of history. The resistance of man against disease changed and so did the external conditions that threatened health. Diseases known as chronic to-day were acute when they first invaded a territory. Geographic and climatic conditions always had a profound influence upon the morbidity of a region. Cultural factors—the mode of living of man, his interfering with the natural rhythm of life, the measures he devised in course of time to fight disease —all altered the health conditions most deeply.

Research in the history of diseases is extremely difficult. The only objective method is the examination of bones and mummies but the material is scanty and is often ill-preserved and difficult to date. Pictures representing morbid conditions may be helpful but one has to be very careful in making diagnoses from pictures. Our chief sources are medical books and documents. Also chronicles, diaries, letters, and novels often contain excellent descriptions of diseases. But it is by no means easy to recognize diseases mentioned in books. If symptoms are striking as in the case of epilepsy, malaria, or gout the task will not be difficult while many other diseases are almost impossible to diagnose from descriptions. Not only has the nomenclature changed but the concept of disease has varied a great deal and the disease entities that we distinguish often do not correspond to those of former periods.

The history of diseases is an extremely important part of medical history. It is its starting point, and without it many medical theories could not be understood. How could we explain the importance attributed in the Hippocratic writings to the spleen—a very inconspicuous organ—if we did not know that the Hippocratic theories were elaborated in regions where malaria was endemic and many people suffered from splenomegaly?

The history of diseases can contribute much to modern pathology and epidemiology. Serious epidemics of influenza occur only once in a generation so that we cannot study the disease without its history. Many other contagious diseases are rare to-day but under special conditions may still become a menace to society. The only way to get acquainted with them is through historical studies. The history and the geography of diseases are most intimately connected and cannot be investigated separately. The problem is to trace the development of a given disease in time and space.

It is regrettable that these studies have been somewhat neglected in recent years while physicians were keenly interested in them during the nineteenth century. August Hirsch's *Handbuch der historisch-geographischen Pathologie* was a masterpiece and has not been surpassed yet.[2] The organization of the Inter-

[2] First published 1860-1864 in 2 vols., 2nd ed. in 3 vols., 1881-1886. English translation, *Handbook of Geographical and Historical*

national Society for Geographic Pathology a few years ago has greatly stimulated research in the geography of diseases, but by neglecting the historical aspect of the problem the Society has deprived itself of a valuable auxiliary.

I once had an ambitious project for a comprehensive investigation of these questions.[3] It was to be started by the foundation of an international journal for historic-geographic pathology that would have served as a clearing-house for all these studies. And it was to be followed by a series of monographs and atlases, each one devoted to the history and geography of a definite disease or disease-group. I had to drop the project because funds were unavailable but I still believe in its soundness and I am convinced that in this particular field historians, by coöperating with pathologists and epidemiologists, could render a valuable service.

Once we are familiar with the incidence of disease at a given period we want to know how society reacted against disease, what was done to restore and protect health. We study the *history of therapy and prophylaxis.* We investigate the history of dietetic, pharmacological, physical, surgical, and mental treatment. It is a relatively easy task. Sources are abundant and their interpretation does not create particular diffi-

Pathology, translated from the 2nd German ed. by Charles Creighton, M.D. (London, The New Sydenham Society, 1883-1886).

[3] "Problems of Historical-Geographical Pathology," *Bulletin of the Institute of the History of Medicine, The Johns Hopkins University,* Vol. I, 1933, pp. 10-18.

culties. A remedy can be prepared from a recipe whether it was written yesterday or a thousand years ago.

Medical literature is our chief source. The majority of all medical books consists of therapeutic treatises. What the doctor needed first of all was instructions on how to treat patients. The oldest medical books, Egyptian papyri and Babylonian cuneiform tablets, contain mostly collections of recipes. Prescriptions and dietetic rules are difficult to remember. Hence they were not transmitted by word of mouth but in writing—sometimes even in verse so as to be remembered more easily. Thus it happens that we can trace the history of the treatment of many diseases almost without gaps.

This is not the case with surgery. Nobody can learn to operate on a patient from books. The surgeon was a craftsman who learned his art while serving a master as apprentice. Surgery therefore was transmitted in a practical way from master to pupil and often from father to son. In many periods of history the surgeons had no general education so that they did not write any books. The fact that there are no written records on the surgery of certain periods does not mean that there was no surgery at all. But then, there were times and countries where the surgeons had university education. These men did write books and it is often difficult to trace the sources of their knowledge on account of the gaps in the history of surgical literature. Where literary sources are missing, instruments, splints, and also pictures may prove extremely helpful.

Special methods have been devised to investigate the history of therapy—methods of experimental archæology. A treatment recommended in former times can be repeated to-day. The efficacy of an ancient drug can be tested in animal experiments. One of my students experimented with medieval anesthetics.[4]

Many ancient treatments discarded for some reason or other by academic medicine survived in folk medicine and are still alive to-day, so that their application and results can be studied in practice. And in many oriental countries, notably in India and China, ancient medicine is still taught and the old classical textbooks are still consulted so that there we can study the history of medicine in life.

Therapy until very recently was mostly empirical. There were theories, to be sure, which seemed to explain the action of drugs and diets. But in many cases the theories were secondary. Drugs were given because they had been applied successfully for centuries before. There can be no doubt that a vast amount of medical experience is hidden in the ancient materia medica. A drug that was found to be efficacious by many generations of physicians cannot be worthless even if we are unable to explain its action in terms of modern science. It happened more than once that

[4] M. Baur, "Recherches sur l'histoire de l'anesthésie avant 1846," *Janus*, Vol. 31, 1927, pp. 24-39, 63-90, 124-137, 170-182, 213-225, 264-270.

a drug was abandoned because medical science had no use for it. And when science progressed and new principles were found the drug was suddenly rediscovered. I think it would be a worth-while undertaking to examine ancient materia medica and dietetics systematically, and without prejudice. It would be a time-consuming piece of research but it might help to improve our own therapy.

The history of preventive medicine is a most fascinating subject that has to be approached from two different angles. The more we know about the cause, nature, and mechanism of a given disease the more efficiently we can interfere in its course, or the better prepared we are to prevent its developing. The history of preventive medicine will, therefore, always reflect the history of medical science. But there is an entirely different side to the problem. It is not enough to know how to prevent disease; we must be able to apply our knowledge, and whether we succeed or fail in this endeavor depends on endless non-medical factors such as the attitude of society toward the human body, its valuation of health and disease, its educational ideal, and many other philosophic, religious, social, and economic factors. Public health measures require a strong administration. The history of preventive medicine is most intimately connected with the general history of civilization.

After having examined the diseases of a given period and the various methods applied at the time to fight them, we would like to know what ideas were guiding society and its medical instruments, the physicians, in their actions. Here we investigate not the craft of medicine but its theory; not the practice of medicine but medical science. Here we make no valuation. Theories were always correct once, until they were superseded when science evolved. Nothing could be more foolish than to compare ancient theories with ours, and to call progressive what corresponds to our views and primitive what is different.

In our previous investigations we needed our medical knowledge badly. But in investigations of theory we must try to forget it, so as not to be prejudiced. All we remember is the external manifestations of disease—its symptoms—and we examine how the physician of different periods saw them, what they thought of them, and what concept of disease they formed. Our choice of sources in this particular field cannot be broad enough because medical science is but one small aspect of general science which, in turn, is part of the philosophy of the period; the result of the general attitude of man toward his fellow men and toward the world at large. A study of the history of art, music, or law can help us to understand medical theories because the general trends that dominated an epoch were expressed in all cultural manifestations.

If we attempt to see the theory of medicine in its cultural setting, then we come to understand why primitive medicine had a magical, and Babylonian medicine a religious, character; why the Greek physicians speculated in terms of philosophy, and the medieval doctors in terms of theology; while after the Renaissance a new medicine based on the natural sciences began to develop. In such light a theory like that of the four humors does not appear fantastic; it was the logical product of the philosophic structure of its time—and besides a very workable theory that explained a great deal. We come to understand why human anatomy flourished in the Renaissance while physiology was a creation of the Baroque mind.

In these studies we will pay due attention to the contributions of the individual physicians, the great doctors who, through their discoveries, advanced medical science and became benefactors of mankind.

The *history of medical ideas* is an important and most interesting subject that can contribute much to the history of civilization. In this field the historian of medicine will have to coöperate very closely with historians of other disciplines.

When we study the history of disease we will soon find that its incidence is determined primarily by the *economic and social conditions* of a society. In all civilizations the rich were less threatened by disease than the poor, for obvious reasons. Poverty of the individual, or of groups, always was the chief cause of disease. Institutions like slavery or serfdom, and developments like the industrial revolution influenced the morbidity of a region most deeply. The mode of production and the working conditions are largely responsible for whether a man's life will be healthy or not. At the time when the French clinic flourished in the early nineteenth century, French workers were slaving for fifteen hours a day in the factories, and received wages just large enough to keep them from starving.

In other words: we must be thoroughly familiar with economic and social history before we can approach the history of disease. And this applies to all other aspects of medical history. Medicine is a social function. There are always two parties involved, the physician and patient, the medical corps in the broadest sense of the word and society. It is not enough to find out what therapies were available at a given time. We have to know whether they were applied or not and to whom they were applied, whether to all the people who needed them, or to the propertied class only. It makes a tremendous difference whether medicine is considered a public service to which every citizen is entitled, or whether the service is sold on a commercial basis to whoever can purchase it. Brilliant as its scientific achievements may be, medicine must fail under such a system once the service becomes too expensive or the population too poor to buy it.

The history of medical ideas is much more closely connected with economic history than is commonly understood. We know what the Renaissance has meant to medicine but we forget that there would not have been any Renaissance if there had not been increased trade which created a strong demand for gold, which in turn started the great sea-voyages that led to the discovery of the world. The idea of medical progress developed from the sixteenth century on because a new economic order was gradually overthrowing the static world of medieval feudalism. The demands of a growing industry stimulated science. New instruments and apparatus were invented. The microscope opened up new horizons to medicine and every improvement of the microscope resulted in new discoveries. The ophthalmoscope inaugurated a new era in ophthalmology, whose entire history is the history of its tools. The X-rays revolutionized medicine.

It is time to break the traditional pattern of medical historiography, and in the book on which I am working at present I am approaching the subject from the sociological angle, writing the history of medicine as the history of human societies in their struggle against disease. Every society produced its food and commodities under a definite system, and as a result had a definite social organization. What were its health problems? What was done to protect and restore the people's health, and how was it done? Once this is established then the part of the individual doctors can be discussed, what they thought, and what they wrote.

The historian first proceeds analytically. He examines sources and analyzes them. Driven by some intellectual curiosity, by a living interest we have attacked a definite problem. In the beginning we had only a vague notion of what things might have been like. While our work proceeded our guesses were confirmed, or we had to amend our views. We squeezed the sources until they revealed their secrets and gradually out of separate elements a synthesis was formed in us. Events, people, theories of the past were resuscitated. Now that we know of them, to us they are alive. And whatever is alive wields influence, an influence that reaches far beyond ourselves because the historian's task is to share his experience with others, to put the result of his researches into words, to give them literary form. Writing of history is a creative process. It is art.

Like every artistic creation a book of history has a strong personal note. It is *my* experience that I am passing on, *my* interpretation of history, what *I* as a result of my labors have come to consider the truth. This is why so much depends on the personality of the historian. The work of a historian of genius will have tremendous persuasive power while the work of a mere craftsman will pass away without any repercussions.

Aristotle is perfectly correct when he says of history: ἔχει τι ποιητικόν, there is something creative, poetical in it. And this is just the reason why history is a powerful instrument of life. True history is always contemporary history, as Benedetto Croce once said, because it is a contemporary interest that drives a man to consult the past. The historian is a member of society. If he is a real historian, conscious of his responsibilities, he will not stand aloof but live in close touch with his fellow men taking an active part in their struggles, sharing their sorrows, their hopes, and joys. Driven by a sometimes conscious but mostly still unconscious urge he consults the past and recreates it in writing history—for his contemporaries.

In the same way the medical historian is a physician living in close touch with the medical problems of his days. But he is not a specialist who perceives only limited aspects of medicine. He endeavors to see medicine as a whole, and not only from the point of view of the medical profession, but of society as well.

This, however, means that medical history is not only history but *medicine* as well. It is part of the theory of medicine. It exerts influence upon the doctors' thinking and, therefore, upon their actions. The medical historian's procedure can be compared to that of the psychiatrist. Just as the psychiatrist by analyzing a patient endeavors to make unconscious complexes conscious so that the patient can face them openly and get rid of them, in the same way the historian by analyzing the past endeavors to make unconscious trends conscious so that we may know of them and may discuss them freely in order to improve conditions.

Medical history teaches us where we came from, where we stand in medicine at the present time and in what direction we are marching. It is the compass that guides us into the future. If our work is not to be haphazard but planful, we need the guidance of history and it is not by accident that all great medical leaders were fully aware of the value of historical studies.

It is a sheer waste of effort to oppose powerful social trends. The historical analysis reveals that these trends are not accidental but the result of the whole economic and social structure of a given society. We can influence developments and can take an active part in shaping the future—there is no reason for fatalism—but we can do so only in certain directions. And history tells us what these directions are.

From all that has been said it became apparent that medical historians bear a heavy responsibility. There are quacks among them and their actions are just as pernicious as those of other quacks. History must be true. True history is always fruitful while pseudo-history is destructive. It is difficult to approach a problem detachedly but the historical research methods impose an iron discipline upon us. Whoever refuses to submit to that discipline and writes history uncritically, or frivolously or so as to prove a thesis, acts like a pseudo-scientist who fakes laboratory reports.

Summing up we can say that medical history is not only the concern of history but of medicine as well. And the medical historian, while serving truth as historian, is endeavoring to contribute to the progress of medicine.

VI

THE HISTORY OF LEPROSY

BY

NEWTON E. WAYSON, M.D.

SENIOR SURGEON, UNITED STATES PUBLIC HEALTH SERVICE

VI

THE HISTORY OF LEPROSY

INTRODUCTION

THE history of a disease of man contemplates its biological evolution or manifestations, and his individual or collective cultural responses to its presence. The former aspect may be considered the particular province of the medical man, but the human reactions to disease are of consuming interest to all. Disease has influenced religious, social, and political beliefs and customs, and they in turn have affected its course, dissemination, and treatment. Battles and wars have been won or lost by it, and men's responses to it have resembled their behavior in battle. If the events of the battle-fields are comprehended they will meet them by fight, but if the unforeseen occurs, or ignorance of the circumstances surrounding the engagement supervenes, they are likely to be overwhelmed by fear and take to flight. They have always been bewildered and frightened by the surprise attack in which the weak and the strong, the young and the old are ravished, and such is frequently the way of disease. Its ruthless onslaughts with invisible weapons have never been understood by them, and they have rushed to their talismen, or importuned their gods for protection, fled in panic, or struck wildly and savagely at those believed to be the perpetrators of the ominous happenings. Fears and superstitions concerning disease have prevailed throughout history, and only their forms and the methods evoked by them have been altered during the different periods. Nor is it correct to infer that inhuman or aimless conduct has been restricted to primitive men of nineteen hundred years before Christ, because the primitive in man is a powerful force nineteen hundred years after Christ, and traditions and folklore are not easily laid aside. Men and races were persecuted, banished, or massacred in olden times because they were diseased, or because of the belief that they were possessed of evil spirits; audiences at the theater, citizens of villages, cities and countries fled in panic from great plagues of the seventeenth century; but "witches" have been murdered and panics precipitated in the United States during the past twenty years.

Bubonic plague, smallpox, cholera, and typhus have struck communities with sudden terrifying force, swept through the entire population with the rapidity of fire, destroyed thousands, scattered other thousands, and left a disordered wreckage of men and manners. They have also vanished almost as quickly and have not returned for generations. Malaria, tuberculosis, and leprosy have advanced more insidiously and have sapped and undermined the people for ages without eruptive outbreaks, but without ceasing. Of these, leprosy has excited the most terror and left the most profound traces on social and political life. It has promoted humanity and hygiene, and precipitated inhumanity and squalor. Nor has the horror of it diminished greatly during our own era. Thus, recently a young woman of high-school education rushed in fright from the laboratory in which she was told that another technician was examining some of the bacteria of leprosy on a glass slide. Again, quite recently, a wedding ceremony between two leprous people in Rumania was conducted by a minister and a clerk who wore long white robes, white gloves and caps, and who after the ceremony hastily withdrew from the scene and burned their garments, and all their accoutrements. Some procedures of the medical staff of a government leprosarium in Japan suggest that they, also, are inspired by fear. Before entering the wards, they don caps, long gowns whose sleeves are fastened around the wrists, rubber gloves and rubber boots, and walk through troughs of disinfectants. Upon returning, the gowns, caps, and gloves are discarded on the ward side of the trough which is forded to leave the boots on the near side of it.

Leprosy has been mentioned in every epoch of history. Has it existed since the dawn of civilization? From whence did it come? Neither its origin, its antiquity, nor its exact prevalence in the past or present is definitely known, and can be only vaguely surmised. The reasons for this lack of knowledge will become more apparent in subsequent discussion, but it may be remarked that statistical determinations of the incidence of disease are not applied with any degree of accuracy to two-thirds of the population of the world of the present day. Thousands who lived in ancient times, and thousands living in the countries of modern civilization have never been attended by trained physicians. Then, too, physicians who have been well versed in the medicine of their own times have confused leprosy with other diseases. How much more likely that priests, princes, burgomasters, barbers, and itinerant charlatans have erred in the diagnosis. Mistakes could not have been avoided so long as the disease was regarded as a visitation of divine wrath or ill-humor, or as the prank or malice of a diabolical spirit, and it is only within recent centuries that even the common fevers have been differentiated. Within the past hundred years typhoid fever was found to be different from typhus, and it is within the lifetime of many that microörganisms were found to be the cause of some affections and at the root of others. Robert Koch discovered the tubercle bacillus only fifty-five years ago, and Hoffman and Schaudinn found the accepted cause of syphilis thirty-two years ago. Until these scientific discoveries were made known, there were no accurate means of separating these two diseases from leprosy, which they frequently resembled, though the bacterium of leprosy was discovered between 1871 and 1874.

The medical historian must project the light of this modern knowledge in retrospect through the centuries in his search of the history of leprosy. He must critically examine pictorial, sculptural, and archæological reproductions, or specimens, and scan the records of court, church, medical institutions, and professional writers. He must at the same time maintain a disposition of scholarly exactitude, and not read into these his personal convictions or imagination. These records and incunabula are often fragmentary, incomplete, and vague. Their interpretations may turn upon the deciphering, derivation, or meaning of ancient obsolete words or colloquialisms. On the other hand, they may be lucid, comprehensive, and freshly descriptive during one epoch, only to be completely lost during another. These handicaps to tracing the origin, prevalence, and migrations of leprosy become even more apparent when the modern concept of it is considered.

DEFINITION

The scientific name of leprosy, lepra, is derived from the Greek word meaning a scale or scaly, and was probably adopted because the formation of scales on the skin is of common occurrence in leprosy. It will be evident that confusion may have taken place with any disease in which the skin produces scales, whether the condition was sunburn or eczema, and, incidentally, some of the manifestations of leprosy do resemble sunburn. The consensus of opinion is that it is a communicable disease caused by a bacterium (*Mycobacterium lepræ*); and that the degree of communicability is slight under most of the circumstances prevailing in the countries of modern civilization.

The manner by which the organism enters the body is not definitely known, but it is believed that it may be introduced through the mucous membranes of the nose and throat, or through either visible or minute wounds in the skin. It is not inherited, but the infants and young children of leprous families are frequently infected; hence, it has been thought, until very recent years, that the infection was congenitally acquired. After the organism has entered the body it may lie dormant through months or years without producing illness, and then slowly, or suddenly, produce recognizable changes.

The first evidence of the infection may be confined to one part of the body, and may be rather insignificant in its appearance or extent, and remain of little consequence for years, or it may spread rapidly to many parts of the skin and nerves. Not all tissues are equally affected, but there is a marked predilection for the nerves, skin, lymph nodes, and bones. An attack may be characterized by acute illness with severe prostration, high fever, skin rashes, or eruptions and swellings, and painful inflammation of the external coats of the eyeball, of the nerves, of the joints and bones. Sensation of the skin is intensified, decreased or lost in most instances, and perhaps in all cases in which the disease is well established. Paralysis may occur during these attacks, or may develop with relative suddenness in one who is affected, but who seems comparatively well. Thus a leprous child who was roller-skating in the afternoon complained during the evening that her legs felt heavy, and on the following morning was found to have a complete paralysis of the muscles of the leg. Progress of the disease may become spontaneously arrested, and the sick individual convalesce to a seemingly normal state of health. Contrariwise, the process is usually a very slow one, and may continue for many years, during which it may progress, recede, or apparently come to an end, or progress continuously by alternately slow and rapid stages. In well-established cases there are usually areas in the skin in which the sensation is diminished or lost for temperature, pain, and touch; the muscles of the face, hands, or feet may become paralyzed and wither; the skin may become thick, hard, and scaly, and may contain pimples, lumps, dark or light spots; ulcers may develop and extend deep into the underlying tissues; bones of the fingers, hands, toes, and feet may be absorbed; the face may become like that of a satyr; the voice harsh or whispering; blindness may occur; and the afflicted individual be reduced to a helpless pitiful state. These late or final changes are those which have been described in older writings, as well as in some of recent date.

ANCIENT HISTORY

The cradle of leprosy has been variously ascribed to the ancient civilizations of Egypt, Babylon, Persia, India, and China. However, the authenticity of its presence among them must be determined solely by the definition or interpretation of words which were provincialisms of the times. The oldest written description of diseases among the Egyptians is contained in the Eber's Papyrus, which dates from the sixteenth century B.C. Several diseases are defined or designated in this by simple names, and one, *uhedu,* has been translated to mean any painful swelling; an abscess; an inflammation of the intestine accompanied by painful joints; and has been interpreted as either syphilis or leprosy. One Egyptologist translates it literally, and another reads into it an interpretative sense. The exhumation and careful examination of a large number of mummies have failed to reveal changes in the bones which are typical of leprosy, and Egyptian statuettes, which were executed with great fidelity to human form, exhibit none of the mutilations which are common to the late or neglected forms of leprosy. However, the people of Egypt were associated with those of other parts of Africa, and of Asia Minor for many centuries in exchanges of trade and through hostile invasion. The Hyksos, a semitic nomadic people of Asia Minor, conquered Egypt in 1700 B.C., and Babylonians, Assyrians, Persians, and others occupied or ruled it during subsequent periods. The geography, climate, and culture of all these people were such as to foster the implantation and dissemination of their respective diseases upon one another. Hence, it becomes difficult to determine which, if any, of these were countries of the original infection.

In ancient writings of India the word *kushta* evidently refers to leprosy, but there is no unanimity of opinion regarding the dates of these records, and authorities seem to ascribe them to a period between the tenth and eleventh centuries B.C., or to that of one to three hundred years A.D. with equally good ground for their respective conclusions. Religion and primitive medicine were inseparable in the thoughts of all the earlier civilizations, and there was close similarity in the measures adopted for the correction of moral or spiritual delinquencies and physical ailments. Both the sinner and the sick were regarded as subjects of divine displeasure. One may wonder whether the grim warning on a stele beside the highway to Babylon five thousand years ago, concerning him who was unclean, and the admonition "Nevermore shall he know the ways of his abiding place" referred to him who was a moral or physical leper. Both interpretations have been suggested. One may also with equal justification accept or reject an interpretation of leprosy in the reference in the Assyrian-Babylonian records to cleansing the spots of the skin of him who has humiliated his flesh, by washing in the waters designated by the boatman of the Master of the subterranean world; or the story of the main warrior of the Syrian King, Benhadad II, who was cleansed of leprosy by bathing seven times in the River Jordan.

Centuries later the great Greek historian, Herodotus (490-420 B.C.) and Ctesias, a famous physician to the king of Persia, cite royal decrees forbidding him who has white spots on his skin from entering the city, and prohibiting the presence of white pigeons, which were also believed to be afflicted with the disease. Likewise, in both old and modern references of India and of Turkestan, the term *white lepra* occurs, but it is impossible to attribute a specific connotation to the term.

The failure to discriminate between different abnormal conditions in which there was a loss of pigment in areas of the skin, such as are of frequent occurrence in those countries, and probably were equally prevalent in olden times, and the conjunction of moral and physical defects in one religious category have made the ancient history of leprosy largely speculative.

BIBLICAL HISTORY

The first acquaintance with leprosy that comes to many in Christian countries is that which is obtained through the teachings of the church and the readings of the Pentateuch. The ancient versions of the Bible use the word "zaraath" in the book of *Leviticus* in which the instructions to the priests are detailed. This word was regarded as synonymous with lepra in the earlier translations when lepra designated a mild superficial skin condition. Translators of later centuries have carried over the interpretation of zaraath as leprosy, which we now know to be a grave and enduring condition of very different character from that described in the Bible. The definition or connotation of this word is made more difficult because of the lack of authentic data for the determination of the period in which the original text was written. The *Septuagint* is supposed to have been written between 284 and 246 B.C. at Alexandria, and is presumed to have reduced to writing the traditions of a scattered people, which had been handed down through the several hundred years since Moses.

It seems certain, also, that the only available manuscripts of the *Pentateuch,* other than fragments, do not date back farther than the ninth century of our era.

A careful comparison of the *Septuagint,* of the *Vulgate of Jerome,* and of later Latin translations of the Hebrew texts attracts the attention to the discordance between zaraath and leprosy. Thus, the priest was admonished to note whether the skin was depressed and contained white hairs. White hairs do not occur in the leprous conditions of the skin. Further, he was to examine the suspect after seven days, and in yet another seven days, and if the condition had not spread and no white hairs had appeared, he was to declare the individual clean, or non-leprous. Leprous conditions of the skin usually change very slowly, and it is very doubtful whether the uninitiated could detect any differences after one or two weeks. There is no mention of a loss of sensation in the skin, nor of paralyses which are of frequent occurrence, nor of the heavy thickened face, the big ears, the reddened or blinded eyes, and the raucous voice, which are common to the advanced or neglected cases which should have been prevalent in those days, if the disease was present. On the other hand, the laws for detection and for cure of zaraath in woolen, linen, skin, or leather garments, and in the walls of houses were equally specific in their application to these inanimate objects. Whereas, leprosy is a disease of human beings. Much doubt is therefore expressed by able and competent scholars concerning the identity of zaraath, or the leprosy of the Bible.

It seems quite probable that the Jewish peoples living on the strip of land between the Euphrates and the sea did have the diseases of the neighboring countries. This land was repeatedly invaded or traversed for centuries by hordes of Babylonians, Assyrians, Egyptians, Chaldeans, Persians, and Greeks who remained in the country for long periods, were quartered on the native people, and again and again enslaved them. Slaves were carried to the countries of the conquerors only to return to their native land even as entire tribes returned from Babylon. The expulsion or exodus of the Jews from Egypt has been attributed to their having as many as eighty thousand cases of leprosy among them, but again there is insufficient evidence for such a conclusion.

GREEK THOUGHT AND THE CHRISTIAN ERA

For ages the misfortunes and illnesses of man were ascribed by him to unfavorable spirits, ghosts, and demons, but about 500 B.C. there was an awakening of thought which directed attention to the natural causes of disease. This philosophy originated among, or was given impetus by, the Ionian Greeks, and persisted for several centuries. Observations were made of the sick man, careful notations were made of his symptoms, and efforts were made to classify his disease and to apply remedies which others had found useful. Records were made during this period of conditions which were unmistakably leprous. While it is now uncertain that ancient Egypt or a country of Asia Minor was the original source of leprosy, it is certain from writings of these Greeks that it existed in these countries between the second century before Christ and the second century of our era. These writers named the condition elephantiasis, and a synonym for leprosy has been *Elephantiasis græcorum* from then until now. The term was probably adopted because of the fancied resemblance of the thickened skin, hanging in folds, to the coarse, loose hide of elephants.

At about the beginning of the Christian Era leprosy had undoubtedly also made its appearance in several other countries bounding the Mediterranean Sea, and particularly in those surrounding its Eastern shores. Pliny the Elder (23-79) stated it was prevalent in Egypt; Plutarch cites d'Athenedorus as authority that it appeared for the first time in Greece between 124 and 96 B.C.; Archigenes (about 100 A.D.) gives an authentic description of it in India. Celsus, who lived in Rome under Augustus and Tiberius Cæsar (27 B.C.-37 A.D.) described it, but he seems to have been greatly influenced by the writings of Pliny, since it was relatively, if not entirely unknown in Italy at the time of Celsus. Pliny states that it was imported by the legions of Pompey. If it was present in Rome, it had not become sufficiently conspicuous or prominent to attract the attention of the law-makers of the second and third centuries who proscribed the sale of slaves afflicted with phthisis, intermittent fever, ophthalmia or mental alienation, but did not mention leprosy.

Assuming the existence of leprosy in Asia Minor for a few centuries before the Christian Era, it is not surprising that it was spread over the remainder of the world, as known at that time, and continued to spread during the next several centuries. Since from the time that Nebuchadnezzar carried the Jews into captivity in Babylon, about 600 B.C., until 50 A.D. when the Roman Empire had reached the zenith of its geographical extent, there were enormous migrations of people in and out of Asia Minor and the countries bounding the Mediterranean. Carthage, Rome, and Alexandria were engaged in feverish commercial activities with one another and with the Near East and the Far East. The armies of Darius, Xerxes, Philip of Macedonia, Alexander the Great, the Scythian hordes, and the Cæsars were marching and countermarching across these countries with thousands in their legions and trailed by other thousands of camp followers and slaves. Women of the conquered were appropriated, or entire populations were transported to the foreign lands as slaves or house-servants only to be recaptured and returned. The Romans carried their campaigns, and, presumably, their diseases into England, Germany, France, and Spain. The Carthaginians were now in Italy, now in England, back in Northern Africa, or sailing down its Eastern coast. The Moors were visitors in Spain, and returned to Africa. Following these five or six centuries of mixing and confounding these peoples of Asia, Africa, and Europe, came another five or six hundred years of swarming of the nomads from the east and southeast of Europe. The Goths, Vandals, and Huns now overran and infiltrated the Roman Empire, so that by the beginning of the seventh century the whole of Europe except the Scandinavian or northern countries had been well seeded with leprosy. The Huns had intermingled with the Mongols, who had penetrated deeply into China.

Leprosy is reputed to have been mentioned in the oldest book of China, dating between 1130 and 250 B.C. One author believes it was present as far back as 1100 B.C. Others date its first presence at about 800 B.C., two or three centuries before Confucius. The nephew of the latter is supposed to have been leprous. In later books (589-617 A.D.) it is comprehensively described under the name of *lei-fou,* and there is some evidence to show that it was prevalent in Southern China and in Cambodia. Japan was settled by people of Chinese origin, and leprosy may have been carried to that country by the ancients or by those of later periods. According to Dohi there is a description of it in the second oldest Japanese law book (702 A.D.), and he believes it to have been endemic in Japan previous to 1100 B.C. However, the oldest leper colony was at Nara near Kyoto, and probably goes back to Queen Gwyo (718-740 A.D), who, by tradition, bathed a thousand lepers with her royal hands. The disease was considered the result of unhealthful air and the entrance of an insect into the body. The Buddhists later dismissed this belief and attributed it to the sins of earlier life.

Toward the end of the ninth century the people of the northlands of Europe had been overwhelmed and crowded back by the Franks and others of the Southern countries, and were forced to take to the seas. Thus arose the famous Viking raiders whose forays became invasions in which seizures of boat-loads of captives were carried off to Scandinavia from these southlands and from the shores of the Mediterranean. During the latter part of the tenth century and the first part of the eleventh leprosy was observed in these north countries, including Iceland and England. An asylum for lepers is reported to have been in England as early as 625. Ireland had one in 889, and Wales one in 950.

CRUSADES

With the beginning of the eleventh century Christianity had become widespread throughout Europe, but a schism had developed between the ecclesiastical and temporal rulers, and a contest for supremacy was waged for years. Emperors regarded themselves as rulers with divine authority, but popes would have none of it, since they looked upon the heads of the Church as the direct agents of Jehovah, and, as such, the rulers of the world. Aspirations for power with divine grace dictated the activities of Church and king. Both were champions of the Lord. In the East, Mohammed had arisen as the self-appointed true prophet of God, and those who were not of Islam were to be persecuted or slain. Wars were carried on between the opposing factions with fanatical fervor in the name of religion, but always at the expense of the devastation of the country and the people. In 1095 Pope Urban II summoned the first Crusade to dispossess the heathen of cities and symbols which were fundamentally of Christian origin, and during the next two centuries great swarms of armed and unarmed mobs deserted homes and lands to tramp with crusading spirit to and fro into Southeastern Europe and Asia Minor. Millions were involved in these migrations, including thousands of children. Thousands returned to their homelands diseased, and afflicted with leprosy. There were no provisions or organizations which were adequate to care for these sick, who were adrift as outcasts and as disseminators of their affliction.

There is ample testimony to show that leprosy was well established and blooming in all Western Europe from England to the Mediterranean and from the Atlantic to Russia long before the summons to the first Crusade, but it flourished during the period of the Crusades and assumed the intensity of an epidemic which lasted until the beginning of the fourteenth century.

LAWS AND CUSTOMS

These century-long marauding expeditions and crusading migrations to and from endemic areas of disease with the resultant collapse of government, and the ruin, devastation, and famine in their wake had made a ripe soil for a harvest of epidemics. Neither were the people, nor their leaders, prepared mentally to meet any general attack of illness. The philosophy of the natural causes of disease which had been evolved by the Greeks had been lost sight of during the Roman conquests, and with the breakdown of civilization during the succeeding centuries there had been a complete reversal to primitive thought. The monastic schools of Charlemagne, who is presumed to have been a great educator, stressed the supernatural in their teachings. The monks were dependent upon the writings of the saints for their knowledge, and these latter were intent upon spiritual matters, and not upon science or natural history. Medicine was in the hands of charlatans, vendors, and quacks. The edicts and decrees of the Church forbade the practise of medicine, but had preserved the medical books in the monasteries. The monk was the only educated man, and the care of the sick was the province of this holy man. He believed that disease was the result of sin or evil spirits; that it was to be controlled by penance and prayer; or by casting out the evil spirits and the banishment of the habitual transgressor, or chronically ill.

Nevertheless some belief of the communicability of leprosy appears to have been continuously harbored from ancient times during all these dark ages and into later centuries. It is mentioned by the ancients, and Avicenna (980-1037), known as "The Prince of Physicians," wrote "that the very air is corrupted as it is in the plague or small-pox, and if contagion can

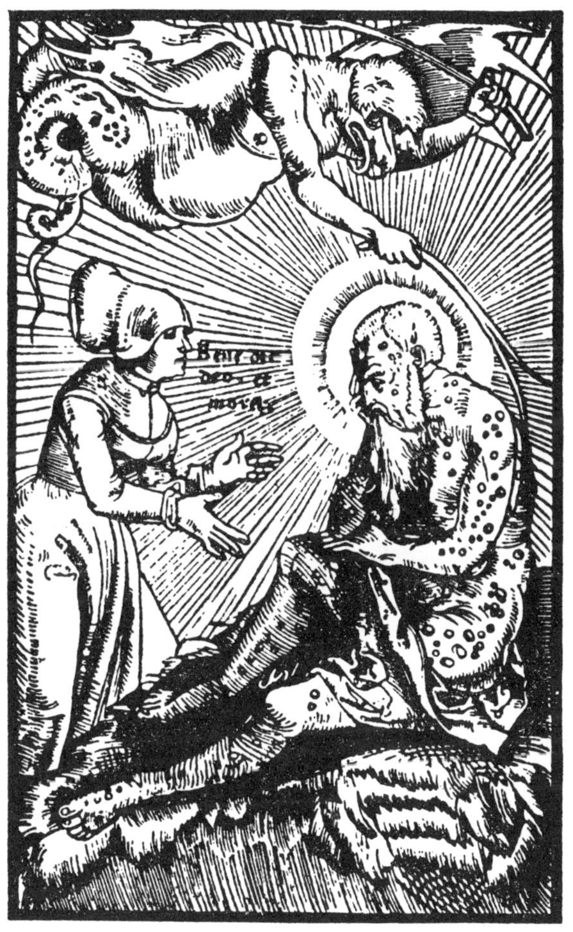

Job, Afflicted with Leprosy (Symbolized by a Dragon with a Scourge), is Exhorted to Patience by a Woman

(After a wood-cut by Hans Wechtelin in *Feldbuch der Wundtartznei* by Gersdorf, 1517)

be propagated this way, i.e., by medium of the atmosphere, in a leprosy how much more active must the venom be in a close and immediate contact."

Efforts towards the suppression of leprosy were made before the Christian era. The supreme resource among these, since the time of Aretæus, has been the isolation of the sick. Kings, prelates, landgraves and mayors issued sporadically their edicts, bulls, decrees, and proclamations to accomplish segregation of the lepers from other citizens or communicants, and to regulate their goings and comings. Rotharo, King of the Lombards (648), decreed the leper civilly dead, and provided for the disposition of his family and his effects. Howel the Good, (tenth century), provided that a son born of a leprous father cannot receive his patrimony, since God has separated the lepers from all their estate here below. The ancient Norwegian laws of Gulathing (tenth and eleventh centuries), exempted the lepers from military service, and authorized the dissolution of the banns of one engaged or married to a leper. Pope Sirice, at the end of the fourth century prescribed that there should be a separation of a clean spouse from a leper, in order that their children should not be tainted. The Council of Compeigne in 757, and the Third Council of Lateran, 1179, issued regulations concerning the marriage of lepers. Charlemagne made provisions for their isolation. The Council of Orleans, 511, the Fifth Synod of Orleans, 549, the Council of Tours, 567, and the Council of Lyons, 583, charged the bishops with duties of asylum and care of the leprous in addition to ministering to their spiritual welfare. Pope Zachary ordered that those who were born leprous must be banished from the city, but might be permitted to beg alms, while those who had acquired the disease were to remain within the city to be cured and were to have communion, but apart from other communicants. Pipin, 757, decreed that leprosy was grounds for divorce. Charles V of France wrote in letters of February 1371: "Since our wars there are large numbers of leprous people coming to our city from foreign lands and from the rural sections of our own country. They associate with our people, frequent the public squares, the streets, the inns, houses of our citizens, and are a menace—therefore all who were not born in the city or do not habitually live here are to take the nearest road to their homeland or to a leprosarium, to which they are to be permitted to enter, under threat of bodily punishment or of fines." This threat was continued in Paris for the next three hundred years, but was honored in the breach. Edward III of England decreed in 1346 that lepers were to be thrown out of the city. A statute of Vincennes prescribed the right of any one to chase the lepers from the city and to beat or despoil them. Special dispensations were made in these various pronunciamentos for those of high estate, who were permitted to isolate themselves, and were admonished to withdraw to rural districts to have good air and food.

Thus a great mass of proscriptions and regimentations had accumulated from the fifth century onwards, but there was no attempt at codification, since there was no political or governmental unity in any of the divisions of Europe. Kings, ecclesiastics, landgraves, and dictators of minor degree were supreme in all the territory they could obtain and hold by divers means. Countries, provinces, cities, and villages each devised and executed their individual practices in accordance with the beliefs of their respective citizens and the prevalence of the disease. All their measures reflected a large element of the conviction of a moral dereliction and fear and ignorance of the scourge. Humanitarian and charitable motives and procedures were interspersed with cruelty and persecution, and occasionally even with massacre. However, in spite of the general discord there were some customs, regulations, and procedures which gradually became common to many districts. These included provisions for the examination of the leprosy suspect, the isolation of the leper, and restrictions relative to marriage, betrothal, cohabitation of spouses, rearing of children, inheritance of family estate, and disposal of personal property.

During the eleventh and twelfth centuries, the civilians who supported some of the leprosaria, and were concerned with the spread of the disease among themselves insisted upon having a voice in the proceedings. Hence, future regulations appear also in municipal ordinances and royal decrees. During the fourteenth century physicians were added to these courts of inquiry, and among them were Arabian doctors who enjoyed the reputation of experts, and who devised more accurate and scientific methods of diagnosis. The famous surgeon, Ambroise Paré (1510-1590), was a member of such a court and his certificates of examination and diagnosis have been preserved. Their comprehensiveness, accuracy, and clarity are remarkably outstanding.

Not all the lepers were apprehended during any period, and the descriptions of those that were brought before the courts are those of advanced cases. A large proportion of the cases were, of course, among the common or poorer people. The register of a court of the sixteenth century shows that suspects examined by the juries were: butchers, bakers, brewers, tailors, keepers of inns, women of easy virtue, and their hostesses. However, neither the highly born, potentates, nor ecclesiastics were spared by the disease. Many of the ecclesiastics who were afflicted became leaders of bands of lepers, and opened or established asylums. Constantine the Great, 323-327, is supposed to have had leprosy. In 770 Pope Stephen III threatened Charles the Great with excommunication should he marry Bertha, a daughter of the King of Lombardy and thereby spoil the blood of the Franks by mixing it with the impure blood of the Lombards. Baudoin, 1173, King of Jerusalem, had leprosy. "One day," said William of Tyr, "the future king was playing with his comrades and fell, scratching his hands and arms. His playmates exclaimed in horror, but the boy made no complaint. His preceptor thought he was displaying bravery and prowess, but the boy stated when interrogated that he felt no pain and that his hands and arms were asleep. He did not resent a bite of his arm made by his preceptor, nor a threshing across his buttocks with a belt." His condition gradually grew worse, he became blind, lost his fingers, and was obliged to renounce his kingship since he could not perform his duties. Henry III, 1574-1589, is reputed to have had leprosy, and was ordered to drink and bathe in the blood of young people for his cure.

The legal procedure which embodied the common practices and which is representative of them can be divided into three sections: the Inquiry, the Verdict, and the Ritual of Declaring the Leper Civilly Dead.

It has been pointed out that the inquiry or examination was conducted by associations of lepers, by ecclesiastics and physicians, and it may be added that entire communities acted as jury and judge from time to time. During later periods investigation became solely the prerogative of the faculty of medical institutions, and professional groups. There was much doleful solemnity surrounding the examinations, and great profundity of knowledge was assumed in gravely applying various tests or signs which were presumed to establish the identity of the disease. The urine and blood were inspected, witnesses were heard, and various spiritual or mythical symbols were consulted. It is probable that the first blood tests of medicine were devised in these examinations; namely, crude oil was poured on the blood, and if after an hour the blood appeared colored, it was considered leprous. In Vivarais the blood of the suspect was collected in a vessel, covered with a cloth and immersed in the fountain of Saint Gengoult. If the blood did not remain red and pure, it was considered to be leprous. With the gradual introduction of informed physicians on these juries or courts, and appraisal of clinical signs in the skin, nose, ears, voice, and bones, and the loss of sensation in the skin, and flesh, the diagnoses became more just and accurate, although the evidence accepted as conclusive was that exhibited by advanced cases.

The verdict was rendered with reference to the degree of development of the disease in the suspect, as follows: (1) The suspect is declared indemnified and is to be certified as not leprous; (2) He is to be admonished that, if he does not adopt a proper hygiene he will become leprous; (3) He is advised to enter a leprosarium; (4) He is afflicted with a confirmed leprosy and should be separated from the well people.

The ceremony or ritual of declaring the leper dead was most lugubrious: The individual was veiled with a black cloth, and kneeled before an altar covered with a black drape. He then heard a mass for him, and upon its conclusion, the priest dropped three pellets of earth taken from the cemetery on his head, declaring, "My friend, this is a sign that you are dead to the world." He added, by way of consolation, "Live in the ways of God." He then read the prohibitions. The leprous person was obliged to change his clothes and don a distinctive costume of the leper. He was furnished a rattle or bell and a begging basket. Thus equipped the unfortunate was conducted to his cabin, whereupon the priest blessed his belongings, and placed before his gate a cross on which was hung a box for alms. The leper was separated from the world. A more cruel fillip was sometimes added to this procedure by forcing the unfortunate one to climb into a grave in simulation of a burial.

The prohibitions were essentially the same in many districts and provinces. They were read with awe-inspiring solemnity in the Church, at the hut of the leper or by the grave in the vulgar language, rather than in Latin, in order that the condemned one could understand them. Examples of these sentences were: I forbid you to enter the Church, the Market, the Mill, the Bakery, and all assemblages of people. I forbid you to wash your hands or personal effects in any fountain or stream of whatever waters they may be, and if you want to drink you are to take the water with your cask or other vessel. I forbid you to go abroad without the habit of the leper, that you may be known to others; nor to be unshod or with bare feet except in your own house." In like manner he was forbidden to touch anything he wanted to buy except with a stick; to enter town or houses; to accept alms in other than his cask or a vessel; to be in company with females other than his own; to travel through lanes or to touch the hedges or bushes by the roadside; to touch children or even to beg from them; and to eat or drink in the company of others than lepers. His marriage or betrothal was dissolved and his children separated from him, and he was dispossessed of his property or it was confiscated. If the wife of a leprous husband elected to cohabit with him, or a husband with a leprous wife, they were both to be conducted to the leprosarium, and any children born to the couple were to be separated from them if they were not marked with leprosy, otherwise they, too, were regarded as leprous.

HOSPITALS AND LEPROSARIA

These prohibitions upon, and banishment of large numbers of sick people necessitated some provision for their asylum and care, and such had been developing in pace with the restrictions on them. Pity and aid had been offered the sick from the time of Christ, whereas they had been formerly universally shunned as possessed of devils. Religious orders and fraternities elected the care and shelter of the poor and suffering as their sole duty and life's work. However, it was not until three to four hundred years after the birth of Christ that hospitals existed for any purpose. A house of refuge for lepers was built by the king of Persia as early as 360 at Cæsarea. The first hospital founded was the Nosocomium of Fabiola in about 460 in Italy, "to gather in the sick from the streets, and to nurse the wretched sufferers wasted with poverty and disease." Interest in the care of the leprous stimulated greatly the building of both hospitals and refuges, and their numbers increased steadily until they were rapidly and largely expanded at the time of the Crusades. In Palestine the Order of Saint Lazarus was founded by Pope Damasius II, as leprosy had spread among the crusaders, and he devoted himself to the care of lepers and other sick. The leader of the Order was frequently a leper himself. St. Francis of Assisi was in charge of the Leprosarium of Gubbio, and the Franciscans, Humiliates, Cruciferæ, and Order of St. George were all active in this work. Royal personages also made a Christian sacrifice by becoming the patrons of lepers or caring for them. Edward the Confessor, Louis VIII, and Louis IX of France, Elizabeth of Hungary, and Katherine of Siena are notable examples. It is reported that St. Francis sent Elizabeth his old coat as a sign of gratitude for her assistance, and tributes to her beneficence have been preserved in painting and sculpture.

Monasteries set aside places of refuge in which the leper could remain throughout his life. Asylums or lazarettos (as they were called) were established in practically every country in Europe. One finds such familiar sites as London, Valencia, Palermo, Malaga, Paris, Verdun, and Metz. It has been estimated that there were several thousand of these refuges during the thirteenth century. During the fourteenth century there were fifty-nine remaining in the immediate environs of Paris.

It is certain that many of these refuges were small and housed one or few persons. Many were huts of primitive construction, but others were of stone or other enduring materials and were used for hundreds of years until they were no longer needed. All were customarily located outside of the cities or villages, in bare fields, on the edge of a watercourse and close to a high-road to facilitate begging, and were surrounded by a palisade. When the community of lepers became large enough, permission was given or orders were issued to them for the erection of more permanent structures for housing, for agricultural utility, and for worship. In some instances, both lands and cattle were allotted to them, and their settlements assumed the appearance of large farms.

The management of the asylums or settlements was left to the lepers or was conducted by members of religious orders. The larger institutions cared for the sick and the poor as well as for the lepers, and there was much intermingling of these classes in both monasteries and hospitals.

The routine in the different institutions varied greatly with their location and the period, but they may be exemplified by the following:

> Each inmate was required to bring his bed. Intercourse with relatives and friends on the outside was prohibited. No mention is made of a doctor; since leprosy was evidently considered incurable and the leper was left to his fate. All intercourse with the healthy was forbidden. If a healthy person from the city must of necessity see an inmate, he was to stand in such a position that the wind blew from the healthy one to the infected one. Probably for this reason the hospital was built on the east side of the city, since there was a west wind. Upon entrance each new patient was required to give a donation —rice, butter, a calf and the like. What the bellman collected in gold, flax, coal, and so on was divided equally daily among the sick. Each inmate had his own room and cellar, free light, and wood for cooking, and there was a heated room for general use or bath. Daily service in the chapel consisted of singing some psalms, and at

meal time there was a repetition. Communion was held every five or six weeks. In the evenings the inmates had to go to bed without a light. The clothing consisted of a linen and a woolen cloak and cap. Every other year they received new clothing.

According to the constitution of Hirschau, a monk with the title of "Spittler" was at the head of the care of the poor and the sick at the monastery. Seven times a year the rooms of the sick were to be swept and the floor to be covered with fresh grass. In every monastery the deacon was to go around once a week, to see if any of the sick were lying about. If he found a man sick, he was to care for him. Should it be a woman, he was to send his servant with bread, wine, or other refreshments. The monastery hospital was given a tenth of all that was given to the monastery in the way of fruits, wine, and so on. The monks ate no meat from four-footed beasts except for health's sake. A tenth of that which grew within the monastery was given to the hospital, and that which was left over on the monks' table after their meal was also given to the hospital. Medical advice was bestowed by the monks, among whom there was always one who had read some medical books, and there were medicinal herbs grown in their gardens.

The leper house in Isaarberg was considered remarkable for the democratic organization of its inmates. The house-master and the house-mistress were chosen from among the sick. Every one was to wear a black or gray cloak without colored lining or trimmings. No one could go out without permission and never was any one to go into beer houses, wine rooms, or other houses. Each one was to have his own spoon, bowl or drinking mug, and bread knife hanging from his belt and was never to use that of any one else. To lie on a bed was prohibited. There was severe punishment for the disobedient. If an inmate should marry either within or without the house, he was immediately separated from the house and could take nothing but his clothes with him. Husbands and wives were separated and were to live quietly, honorably, and decently.

Begging days were set aside and each had to take his turn on the roads or in the city. Certain foods such as pork, and dried and old herrings were considered harmful and were interdicted. Treatment was administered in some of the institutions, and the following is the recipe of a pious Sister: One was to take a bath with a decoction of Agrimonia, Hysoppus, and Asarum to which had been added menstrual blood in sufficient quantity. After the bath one was to grease one's self with goose fat and hen fat.

Other remedies whose potency was equally doubtful were used, but the above is characteristic of their bizarre and complex constitution.

DECLINE OF LEPROSY IN EUROPE

During the twelfth and thirteenth centuries leprosy apparently reached the height of its incidence, and through the succeeding centuries it has steadily declined. Neither the number of lepers, nor the number of leprosaria can be estimated with much accuracy. Many lepers were never recognized nor apprehended when known, and all traces of hundreds of leprosaria have been irretrievably lost. During these periods several famines occurred, and people were forced to eat spoiled rye on which the fungus of ergot had grown. Thus, ergot poisoning, known as St. Anthony's fire, was produced in epidemic intensity. This poison causes disturbances in the circulation of the fingers and toes as well as in other parts of the skin, and the fingers and toes may shrivel so that they become dead.

Erysipelas, which was doubtless included as St. Anthony's fire, was also exceedingly common and was spread through hospitals, monasteries, asylums, and jails. Both of these conditions were mistaken for leprosy, and the afflicted ones were accepted as leprous. The records which are at hand of the more permanent institutions indicate that they were gradually deserted or turned to other purposes, including the care of the tuberculous, from the fourteenth century forward.

To-day there are but few cases in Europe and many of those are imported from the colonial possessions. The reasons for the decline are very likely complex, and attempts to denote them have led to several hypotheses and speculations. Social and economic affairs were changing, the great pilgrimages had ceased, and a tremendous flare of commerce was again in progress. During the first part of the fourteenth century, in 1348, the plague of the Black Death slew thousands in the cities and countrysides of the whole continent. Some scholars estimate the mortality of this epidemic at twenty-five million. Smallpox and typhus raged in epidemics and killed their thousands, and it seems probable that all these scourges fell heavily upon the poor and the leprous. Population was thinned out in both homes and cities, and the crowded conditions were mollified. Work was more

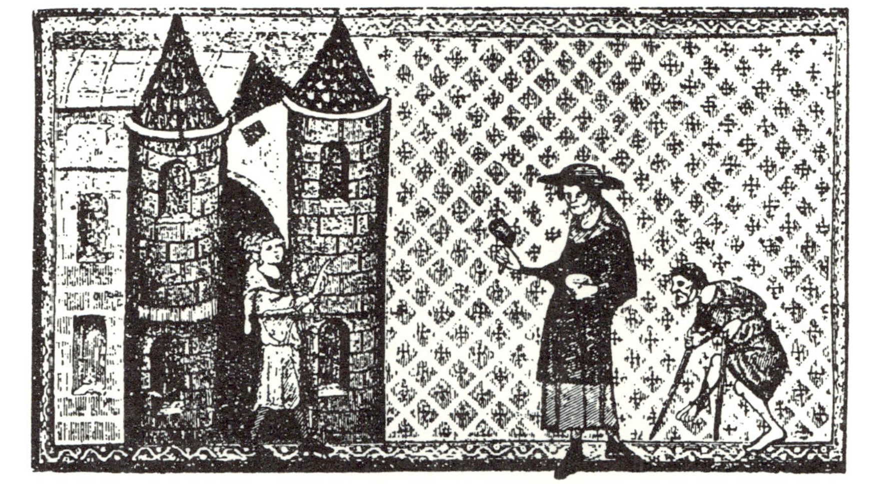

Leper at the Gate of a Medieval City

(After a twelfth-century miniature in the Bibliothéque de l'Arsenal)

plentiful for those remaining alive, and wages became higher. There was also a gradual renascence of medicine, and it was recognized that, aside from ergot poisoning, other chronic diseases such as syphilis and tuberculosis were being mistaken universally for leprosy.

The food of people in England during the fourteenth century consisted of black bread, rye, and salt fish. Salt fish was stored and hoarded. It was used for the *pièce de resistance* in formal banquets among the well-to-do, and was left as legacies to the poor. There was no corn; gardening was not practised; agriculture was but poorly understood; and, of course, there was no manner of preserving foods through the winter except by curing. Gardening was introduced in England in 1509, and hops, salads, turnips, potatoes, tobacco, and tea came during the sixteenth century. After the Black Death there was a great decline in the use of salt fish, and the contemporaneous decline in leprosy was attributed to this latter.

Better food was coming slowly, personal hygiene was improving, people were somewhat cleaner, and there was some attempt at sanitation and better housing. It is necessary to recall the standards and customs of living during the era of the greatest prevalence of leprosy to appreciate how conducive they were to the spread of any communicable disease. The bed of the house was a wooden trough or box arrangement of about six to twelve feet square, covered with a pallet on which the entire family slept in the nude. Straw was first used for the king's bed in England in 1242.

The wayfaring stranger or guest was taken into the same bed with the family. Those who possessed a shirt, a rare occurrence, removed it, rolled it up, and used it as a pillow. Such beds were also in common use in the hospitals, and no effort was made to separate those patients with communicable conditions other than the itch. The inns were incubators of disease, and harbored many escaped or itinerant lepers as well as other multitudinous vagrants. The artisans or servitors had more crowded quarters, and slept on straw or stubble which was covered with a thin cloth. Thus, they were subjected to the pricks of the sharp straw, as well as to those of the swarms of creatures in the straw. The later substitution of cotton or linen underclothing was a progressive advance over the use of woolen garments which were seldom if ever washed, became foul with sweat and dirt, and were the ideal harbors of lice and other parasites which thrive in such habitats. The public baths were open to the leprous vagabonds as well as to all others. Eating habits were primitive. The common bowl into which all dipped, wiped, or messed was universally used. Forks were scarcely known in royal households until the sixteenth century. Soup was poured into troughs hollowed out of the wooden table-tops, and was scooped or lapped. Table wastes which were dropped to the earthen floor remained strewn amongst the straw or rushes which covered the floor. The convivials passed around the flowing bowl from one to another. The host who was entertaining select or notable guests drank first from the common cup and passed it around from one to another of the assembled banqueters. Nobles were served their food on a big square of bread which could be used as a mop or napkin. Later they were served on earthen or metal platters.

The rivers were the sources of drinking water, and also served for the disposal of sewage or waste deposited in them or washed in by the rains and surface waters. Human excrement was deposited on the ground or reached it by discard from upper windows. In 1349 the streets in England were so abused with lay stalls that a proclamation was made "that no person whatever should presume to lay dung, guts, garbage, offal, or any other odure in any street, ditch, or river, upon penalty of £20."

Glass was uncommon in windows, and these were not indulged in extensively since there was a tax on them. Lighting was by candle, or by torches on the highways and in public places.

The streets were unpaved, narrow, and served the hogs as wallows, as well as man and cattle as runways and highways.

Improved economic conditions, the development of community sanitary methods and the restriction of immorality and promiscuity in personal habits have apparently served to limit the spread of several diseases, and it seems likely that they may also have assisted in the disappearance of leprosy.

At all events the incidence of the disease declined sufficiently during the latter part of the seventeenth century, and became so rare in some districts of the country during the eighteenth that the celebrated Danish physician Hensler, professor of medicine at the University of Kiel, was perplexed over the diagnosis in a patient who presented himself, and appealed to a noted colleague of Amsterdam, who replied that he had not seen a case of leprosy during forty years of practice.

DISTRIBUTION IN WESTERN HEMISPHERE AND ISLANDS OF THE PACIFIC

However, the ship physicians were familiar with it, since it was prevalent in the colonial possessions in the Americas and in Oceania. Ships had been plying between these outlying territories and Europe with increasing frequency for two hundred years. Colonists were transported in large numbers, and cargoes of millions of Africans were shipped to ports scattered over the Americas to work as slaves on the plantations and as body servants. The natives of these new lands seemed to be virgin material for the implantation of the diseases of the old countries and leprosy became firmly established. It has flourished in North and South America, and in the islands lying in the Atlantic and in the Pacific on the trade routes between the continents since the early part of the nineteenth century. The records of old explorers are silent concerning its presence in South America during the conquests of that continent. Cortez founded a leprosarium in Mexico during the early years of his dominion, but it was subsequently closed, and another reopened in 1572. During the seventeenth century leprosy was reported in Brazil. The first cases in Colombia are stated to have been observed in Spaniards. It was known to the Maoris in New Zealand for a long time, and probably for centuries, because Captain Cook found it prevalent, and the Maoris had ceased their long journeys during the latter part of the fourteenth century. It seems to have been prevalent in the Philippines during the sixteenth century. The first official register of a case in Canada was in New Brunswick among French people who had originated in an area in Normandy in which it was endemic. There is some speculation as to its origin in Louisiana in the early years of the nineteenth century. Some investigators hold that it was introduced by the migrations of the French from Tracadie to Louisiana, and others that it was brought in by the African slaves. Leprous beggars are supposed to have plied the streets of New Orleans in such numbers as to compel the city fathers to establish a lazaretto in 1785.

Much debate has arisen over the possibility of its presence in the Americas previous to the coming of Columbus. The reproduction of mutilated hands and faces on human figurines in old pottery, and the discovery of diseased bones has led to the assumption that leprosy was present among the primitive people of the country. It has been pointed out with equal cogency, however, that these findings may be indications of other diseases. Furthermore, the readiness with which leprosy spread among the natives with the coming of the Europeans, and its absence among those natives who did not come in contact with these newcomers are rather convincing rebuttals of this reasoning.

DEVELOPMENTS OF NINETEENTH AND TWENTIETH CENTURIES

During the Renaissance all medicine made much progress, and the study and classification of disease were advanced markedly, but the renewal of interest in the study of leprosy was instituted by the Norwegian physician, Daniel Danielssen and his assistant, Carl Boeck, of Königsberg. In 1839 these men began an exhaustive study of the history of the disease in England, Scandinavia, and several other countries of Europe from north to south and east to west. They conducted painstaking observations of the different types of cases, made studies with the microscope and published the results of their investigations in a treatise which affords much of the foundation of the current knowledge of the subject. They were convinced, however, from their observations and from unsuccessful attempts to reproduce the disease by inoculation that it was hereditarily transmitted, and they emphatically denied its communicability. They ascribed its development to faulty ways of living, including defective ventilation, the consumption of raw fish and certain sea birds, and to other unsanitary practices. The Norwegians lived in their houses with their animals under the same roofs, and with doors and windows tightly closed against the long severe winters even during the time of Danielssen and later.

A few years later a German pathologist, Rudolph Virchow, described the microscopic or cellular changes which occur in the leprous tissue. In 1874 Gerhard Hansen published a description of little brown clumps of bacteria which he found repeatedly in the peculiar cells discovered by Virchow. The observations, classifications, and discoveries of these four men in the early part of the nineteenth century have established the first definite and scientifically accurate criteria by which the disease can be distinguished. Sir Jonathan Hutchinson, a noted English pathologist, had popularized the theory of the eating of raw fish as the cause of leprosy, and he clung to his ideas for a long time after these discoveries had shown his hypothesis to be untenable. In fact, it is reported that he was convinced of his fallacy by observations that he made of natives of the interior of Africa who abstained from the eating of all fish because of a religious taboo, but who were nevertheless affected with leprosy.

Though Hansen's findings have been repeated by many investigators throughout the world, it has been impossible to grow the bacterium within the laboratory. Many have believed they have succeeded, but their results have not been accepted by other competent students of the subject. A great handicap in establishing the proved identity of the bacteria grown by numerous investigators has been the universal failure to reproduce the disease in animals with these cultivated bacteria. Many species of the lower animals have been inoculated with the cultures and with leprous material taken from patients, but to no avail. Any one of several animal species will develop a lump and ulcers at the point of inoculation, but the disease has not developed in the animal. Tests have been made on men which have also been inconclusive. Researches have been made to discover the route by which the organism enters the body; whether insects will carry the virus; whether contact with earth which harbors bacteria resembling that of leprosy will produce the disease, but convincing results are yet to be obtained.

Though lacking all these fundamentals to a scientific approach to treatment, efforts have been made for years to find a drug or drugs which will effect a cure. Many remedies have been tried, but one which has been the subject of much notoriety is that of chaulmoogra oil. This oil has been used probably for several centuries in the orient because of a legendary tradition that a leper withdrew to the forest, ate the nuts of the tree from which the oil is derived, and returned cured. The tree is indigenous to East India, and the oil is prepared by pressing the nuts. Both the oil and several refinements of it have been used for a number of years, but it is no longer believed to be a specific remedy. Some patients grow progressively worse while taking it, and others improve, but the same course takes place without the use of the oil. However, the persistent efforts of students of the subject have evolved methods of treatment which have undoubtedly assisted in the arrest of the disease in many patients, and perhaps have effected their permanent convalescence.

During the twentieth century there has been an increasing interest in the subject and national or international bodies or associations have fostered and stimulated investigations in many parts of the world. General Leonard Wood became interested in the care and relief of the large number of leprous in the Philippine Islands while he was Governor-General, and the people of the United States subscribed a fund as a tribute to him and his work for the establishment of a memorial foundation for the study of leprosy. This is known as the Leonard Wood Memorial or the American Leprosy Foundation. The British Empire Leprosy Relief Association, the American Mission to Lepers, a committee of the Health Section of the League of Nations, and the International Leprosy Association are representative groups which are at work on the problem to-day.

Leprosy is still present in all sections of the world; in high or low altitudes, in the cold, temperate or torrid zones, on the seacoast, or inland. It is very prevalent in some parts of Asia, Africa, South America, and in islands of Oceania and the Antilles. In Europe and the Northern part of North America it is relatively rare, but remains in Southern states and Mexico. In the Hawaiian Islands, in the Philippines, and in the West Indies where life practices among some natives are as promiscuous and unsanitary as they were in Europe during the twelfth and thirteenth centuries, there are many cases in proportion to the respective population. The number of cases in continental United States is unknown, and many of those known are imported from other countries. About four hundred of these are under the care of the United States Government in a thoroughly modern institution in Louisiana. The Federal government is also conducting scientific investigations in Hawaii in coöperation with the Territorial government which maintains and controls a leprosarium. The government of the Philippines maintains a settlement of about six thousand cases on a single island of the Archipelago.

The principles of the laws and regulations of the dark and middle ages are still in effect in many countries including the United States possessions. The examinations of the leper-suspect are carried out by a jury of physicians of presumed skill in the diagnosis, and their decision is final. One who is certified to be leprous in Hawaii and in the Philippines must enter a leprosarium. In continental United States, and in other countries in which for one reason or another it is impracticable to make the isolation in a leprosarium mandatory, there is a system of voluntary commitments. In several countries it is not practicable to care for more than the helpless cripples and indigents. Leprosy remains a cause for divorce in Hawaii, and the children of leprous parents are separated from them. The execution of the measures is perhaps more humane than formerly, and in Hawaii, in the Philippines, and in continental United States the leprous people receive care which is far superior to that which they are able to command in their ordinary walks of life. In Hawaii and in the Philippines they live in a segregated district of an island and carry on their lives in just the same manner, and with more modern conveniences than they would in one of their respective villages. They are furnished with churches, houses of entertainment, and stores. They conduct their own courts and other civil procedures. They can marry within the leprosarium and live as husband and wife in their own homes. Theirs is a life in Hawaii which they would regard as a Utopian socialism, since they do not work or have a care for their physical welfare. The government furnishes all. There are more automobiles privately owned by the lepers than obtains in any other village of equal size in the islands, and the same may be said of savings accounts.

SUMMARY

In summarizing it may be said that the accounts of the origin of leprosy and its presence in ancient and biblical times are vague and indefinite. Beginning with the Christian era it was known to be present around the littoral of the Mediterranean and has spread over the entire world as known in the various epochs of history. It appears that where man is, there is leprosy. Its dissemination has been intimately connected with the migrations, explorations, and conquests of the world, and thus its history suggests that it is a communicable disease of humans. The manner of caring for those afflicted has varied with the culture and philosophy of the times, and has reflected fear and horror of it. The principles of its control have been much the same for the past thousand years, but the interest and effort of groups who are making scientific investigations of leprosy offer a hopeful outlook for its suppression.

VII

THE STORY OF THE GLANDS OF INTERNAL SECRETION

BY

WALTER TIMME, M.D.

PROFESSOR OF CLINICAL NEUROLOGY, COLLEGE OF PHYSICIANS AND SURGEONS, COLUMBIA UNIVERSITY

VII

THE STORY OF THE GLANDS OF INTERNAL SECRETION

THERE are scattered throughout the body a number of small masses of tissue each of whose function it is to produce one or several highly important secretions. The secretions consist of powerful biochemical substances which are given to the blood stream or other circulating media to be distributed to the body generally, and by their action to maintain the normal activity and reactivity of the entire organism. Therefore all life and its continuity depend upon them. Because they give off their products directly to the circulation they are known as the glands of internal secretion as distinct from those glands that deliver theirs through the medium of a duct or channel. Hence they were also known as the "ductless" glands. But it was then discovered that some of the glands with ducts had an internal secretion in addition—such as the pancreas and the testicle—and the name "glands of internal secretion" or "incretory glands" was substituted. Their number is still somewhat in doubt because of the lack of unanimity among investigators in recognition of the specificity of the secretions of a few of these structures.

Even in ancient medicine were the results of disturbances in these glands recognized, and measures taken to correct them:

"There are three fundamental principles underlying and maintaining a healthy equilibrium of the body, namely, nerve force, metabolism, and the regulation of heat and mucous and *glandular secretions*." This statement is not, as you may think, of modern origin but dates back to Hindu medicine ten centuries before the Christian era. The three terms used by the Hindus to express these conditions were *vayu, pitta* and *kapha*. They recognized many of the clinical features of disturbances in bodily constitutions which we now know as due to abnormal changes in the glands of internal secretion, and made practical use of their knowledge. Thus they sought to avoid old age with its failings by increasing the virility of the organs by utilizing many of the herbs and concoctions the nature of which has not been handed down to us. They recognized the changes that take place in pregnancy, the pigmented areola around the nipples and the greater prominence of hair on the body. They prohibited their high caste devotees from marrying certain types of women—those particularly with much hair on the face and a nasal brow, for they knew that this type was not fruitful. Red-haired females likewise were more or less taboo for their unbridled temper and uncoöperativeness. There were mixed with these truths many queer and curious misconceptions. They believed for instance that semen is produced in every part of the body, which is not true, and collected at the base of the bladder, which is. They thought that if conception occurred on the unequal days of the menses that the child would be a female, otherwise male—but this was merely a guess and a bad one, for conception does not occur during menstruation at all. But we to-day, as yet, cannot as far as the infant's sex is concerned, make a true one.

The milk found at the end of pregnancy was due, the Hindus thought, to the cessation of the menstrual flow and its determination to the breasts instead of to the vagina. The Laws of Manu, the early Aryan codified rules of conduct for these early peoples, give us an insight into their marvelous conceptions of life and development and death and their means of accommodating themselves to these conceptions. They were preëminently thinkers and not doers and among us to-day are recognized the same type of human who can construct our universe along lines which his theory tells him ought to be correct, but which generally fail when brought into rough contact with fact. They were the prototype of our arm-chair philosophers. And so their ideas of the internal secretions based upon long experience and observation, though the first recorded in history, are subject to anatomical and physiological correction.

The Hindus used a decoction of bucks' testes in milk for energy production, called *kawa-soutra,* and they also treated impotence with testicular tissue. It is also interesting to know that the Chinese used powdered placenta for postpartum hemorrhage.

When we come to their successors, the Greeks, we again are confronted with thinkers and a priori reasoners, but with practically no background of experimentation. Hippocrates, 460 B.C. is the outstanding advocate of this school. They thought that disease was due to the deficiency or absence of some unknown substances which the body required. And as the body is made up of individual organs, the diseases of these organs could be mastered by giving the patients, as medicine, preparations of these organs made from animals. Thus in liver diseases, they gave wolf's liver, in diseases of the chest and respiratory organs they gave fox lung, and of greatest importance—for impotence, they gave sex-gland material.

Celsus and Diosconides—Roman physicians in the first century of the Christian era, employed this method of treatment regularly. It was known as "opotherapy"—the treatment of disease with juices. (Greek—ὀπός, juice). Shortly after them Pliny described swellings in the throat (goiter) caused by drinking noxious waters; and furthermore prescribed testes of donkeys and stags for sexual stimulation. Then for several centuries came isolated descriptions of thyroid disturbances and their cure. The Chinese possibly used thyroid gland in the treatment of myxedema, which we now know as a thyroid deficiency disease. The Byzantine Aetius gave the first recorded description of goiter in 500 A.D. and curiously enough there is described a cure of goiter credited both to Roger, a surgeon of Palermo, and to Arnaldus Villanovanus of the twelfth century with the use of burnt sponges and seaweeds—both known to contain comparatively large amounts of iodine.

And so we see in closing the chapter of ancient medicine that many facts are beginning to stand out as well as theories that deal with the internal secretions. The thought, so frequently expressed, that internal glandular medicine is the newest of the medical specialties is not warranted. It is actually among the oldest. Apparently many of the materials derived from animal tissues needed some further modification to make their cures more definite and of longer duration, for as we approach the Middle Ages we see that not only are the crude medicaments heretofore utilized still in favor but many of their finer qualities are brought into play by the proper incantations, the proper broths, the proper excipients. And curiously enough, the ordinary animal world was not sufficient for the necessary crude basic material out of which were fashioned the newer, more elegant preparations, so our predecessors must needs go to the human body for fresh pharmacopœial delights. And as their patients, or rather victims, were men, so they began to think that possibly medicaments and drugs made from the bodies of men would prove more beneficial and more specific than if made from animals. And so nails and hair and saliva and milk and menstrual blood and urine and even dung were all used. And not content merely with these, they resorted to extracts made from human dead, indeed, even mummies. This filth pharmacopœia of the Middle Ages had no limits in the materials it utilized from all parts of the body, all extravagantly prepared with the utmost care and concern. What interests us chiefly in this period is that the basis for these medicaments seems to have been the theorem of Paracelsus that heart cures heart, spleen spleen, lungs lung. And so we find in the London pharmacopœia of the seventeenth century the statement that "experience has found that human semen is good against the imbecility of the Instruments of Generation and some use it to make a magnetik mummy of to serve as a Philtron to cause Love." The following, taken from a London pharmacopœia of the sixteenth century cites one instance of the preparation of human tissue for pharmaceutical use:

> Artificial, or Modern Mummy:—take the carcase of a young man (some say red-hair'd) not dying of a Disease but Killed; let it lie 24 Hours in clear Water in the Air, cut the Flesh in pieces, to which add Powder of Myrrh, and a little Aloes: Imbibe it 24 Hours in the Spirit of Wine and Turpentine, take it out, hang it up twelve Hours; imbibe it again 24 Hours in fresh Spirit, then hang up the pieces in a dry Air and shady place, so will they dry and not stink.

Out of this they made tinctures, elixirs, balsams and what-not. Interesting in this connection is to read that the secundines (or the after-birth) is recommended to cure struma (or goiter), the falling sickness (or epilepsy), and causes the dead child to come away (uterine contractions). This comes close to some of our modern treatments. But in the early eighteenth century under the influence of cynical and clear-headed, unafraid physicians, this filthy pharmaceutical method was abandoned.

In the meantime the anatomists began to give us real knowledge in the matter of the internal glands. These glands of internal secretion, because they had no ducts or channels to take their manufactured products into the circulation, were known as the "ductless" glands. But in recent years, because some of the glands with ducts, such as the pancreas or the testicles, were also known to give a secretion directly to the blood stream and used their ducts merely as a channel for their better-known products to be directed where they were needed, the term ductless glands was discarded for the more comprehensive term, "glands of internal secretion." Vesalius in 1543 described and named the pituitary gland although it was known to Galen in the second century A.D. as was also the thyroid. Vesalius also described the thyroid in 1543 and Wharton particularly in 1656 who gave it the name, thyroid. While the existence of the thymus gland was probably known to the Greeks it remained for a Swiss physician, Felix Plater, in 1614 to publish an autopsy report of an infant which had died from suffocation by an enlarged thymus gland, a *mors thymica*—quite a modern conception. The suprarenal glands were described in 1563 by Eustachius and named by a Frenchman, Riolanus, in 1628. Not only were the anatomists engaged in these studies, but many interesting correlations of disease of the glandular mechanisms with symptoms began to appear. Thus in 1705 Raymond Vieussens stated that epileptiform seizures were associated with pituitary disease in the case of a prominent Cardinal treated by him.

Even at this day the connection between some forms of epilepsy and pituitary disease is recognized and many papers by prominent physicians are in evidence. In 1761 de Haen associated amenorrhœa—a lack of menstruation—with pituitary disease; and the most modern theories of the anterior lobe of the pituitary gland agree with this statement. The famous John Hunter of London experimented in 1762 with transplants of testes into fowls noting their effect on the secondary sex characteristics. But it remained for a Frenchman, Theophile de Bordeu, to present for the first time in 1776 a clear statement of the function of the glands of internal secretion. He published the doctrine that each gland or organ produces a specific substance which is passed into the blood and that the entire organism is dependent upon these specific substances for its maintenance. This is the idea expressed by the modern term *hormone,* derived from the Greek ὁρμάνειν meaning, "I excite." That is to say, a hormone excites other tissues of the body to maintain their activity. Bordeu also described the bodily changes that take place in eunuchs, capons and spayed females as a result of the deprivation of sexual secretions.

THE THYROID GLAND

It might be well at this point to indicate the gradual trend of medical thought by taking up the discussion of the thyroid gland. (Thyroid from the

Greek θυρεός, shield.) Even the Romans knew that endemic goiter existed in the Alps and it is mentioned both by Juvenal and Pliny. Goiter as you probably know simply means a swelling of the thyroid gland. Paracelsus in the sixteenth century recognized endemic goiter in Salzburg, Austria, and attributed it to the mineral constituents of the water. Interesting to note is the fact that he associated cretinism with goiter. And the use of iodine in goiter, mentioned before, was possibly known to the early Chinese as it was certainly in the Mediterranean regions as early as the twelfth century, for they used burnt sponges and seaweed, both charged with iodine, in its cure. Of course, they did not know the particular ingredient of the ash which accomplished the result. But it remained for several European physicians to describe goiter, during the first half of the nineteenth century. The Englishman Parry collected eight cases of the disease up to 1815. The findings were published in 1825, ten years after his death. But while he described them fully, he did not affix a name to the malady and hence the honor of the discovery seems to have passed him by. It is much like the discovery of America with the name-labeler, Amerigo Vespucci, carrying the honor instead of Columbus. In 1835 Robert Graves of Dublin published a classical description of exophthalmic goiter with especial reference to the exophthalmos, the bulging of the eyes; and in 1840 Basedow, a German physician, described the cardinal symptoms of the disease so thoroughly that, at least in Germany, it has been ever since called by his name—Basedow's Disease. The three symptoms were: the thyroid swelling, the eyeball protrusion, and the rapidity of the heart. Earlier in the century, 1802, an Italian—Flajani—described a condition called *bronchocele* in which goiter and rapidity of the heart were combined. The Italians consider him the discoverer and so in Italy the name of *morbo di Flajani* is pinned to exophthalmic goiter. England and America, when using a name for the disease invariably turn to Graves. And so we have Graves' Disease, Basedow's Disease and Flajani's Disease, depending upon one's patriotic predilection. Parry is all but forgotten.

To go a step further in thyroid history, the first excision of the thyroid was performed by Theodore Kocher of Berne, Switzerland, in 1878. Within four years he discovered that 30 per cent of his cases suffered from a cachexia following the operation, that is to say, from a progressive decline in health, to death in many instances. Reverdin of Geneva a year later showed death to be due to the loss of thyroid function by the complete removal of the gland.

Maritz Schiff of Frankfort completed the explanation when he showed that although all his dogs with thyroid removal died of cachexia, yet if he grafted thyroid tissue beneath their skin, or gave thyroid juice, or raw thyroid by mouth after the operation, the dogs survived. In 1891, G. R. Murray of London recognizing that myxedema (the name given to the disease caused by deficiency of thyroid activity) was one form of thyroid deficiency, gave a woman patient thyroid both by mouth and subcutaneous injection. She improved and lived until a few years ago. Sir William Osler, in reporting the successful use of thyroid by oral administration in myxedema wrote that "not the magic wand of Prospero or the brave kiss of the daughter of Hippocrates ever affected such a change." To-day these various steps seem far apart and long drawn out, but it simply goes to show how slowly, methodically, judicial, logical advance is made. But well made, it rests permanently upon solid foundations.

The next step in the thyroid evolution is to determine what the important ingredient is that produces so many important consequences—positive by its presence—negative by its absence. Many investigators have taken up this problem. At one time it was thought that the iodine content of the thyroid was its most important constituent, but iodine alone in animals deprived of their thyroid is not efficacious in the restoration from their cachexia. After many years of trial, it was finally determined by E. C. Kendall of the Mayo Clinic in 1914 that there is an active principle in the thyroid gland which he extracted in an exceedingly pure state and which he believes to contain all the properties of thyroid extract. This hormone he called *thyroxin*. It is interesting to note that the discovery was almost accidental. As Kendall himself told it to me, the following is his report of the discovery:

At the time of the first tests I returned to the laboratory one evening and dissolved some material from the thyroid which contained about 48 per cent of iodine, in absolute alcohol. The object was to see whether the material could be crystallized from alcohol after it had been concentrated to a small volume. The beaker containing the solution was placed on a steam bath and I sat down at the desk to wait until the solution had concentrated. After a short interval I fell asleep and remained asleep for about thirty minutes. When I looked at the beaker, not only had most of the alcohol evaporated but it had gone to dryness and in the bottom of the beaker there was a white crust on which there was a small amount of brown oily material. It did not look promising so I decided to add more alcohol and reconcentrate in the hope that it would crystallize. The addition of alcohol quickly demonstrated that the oil was still soluble in the alcohol but that the white crust was insoluble. This was removed, and since partially pure thyroxin was so easily soluble in alcohol it seemed probable that this white material was an impurity which should be discarded. Before doing this however I determined its percentage of iodine and found it to be 60. This proved to be almost pure thyroxin which had become insoluble in alcohol and had crystallized from the very small volume just prior to the evaporation of the last traces of alcohol. Had I remained awake, I would undoubtedly have stopped the evaporation before the crystals had separated and the effect of this on scientific progress can readily be seen.

However, the importance, nay, even the necessity for thyroid activity of the presence of iodine is well recognized. There are certain regions in the world in which there is a marked lack of iodine in the soil, the water, and the atmosphere. Throughout these regions many individuals develop, as a result of this lack, inadequate thyroid activity. As a consequence, the thyroid gland, unable to furnish thyroxin to the body, retains its secretions and becomes a boggy, enlarged mass. This is seen as goiter, and does not mean an overactive thyroid as many supposedly believe, but an underactive one. The regions in which such goiters appear in this country embrace, going from East to West, the upper Hudson Valley, to Lake George and Lake Champlain, thence along the Mohawk River through Central New York State and involving the Lake Districts clear to Lake Ontario and Lake Erie including all the towns and cities, and including Rochester and Buffalo. Then it follows the Great Lakes across Ohio, Michigan, Indiana, Illinois and Wisconsin. All the cities in these states, especially along the shores of these lakes, are involved. Detroit, Cleveland, Toledo, Chicago are all affected. Then there is a slight diminution of the incidence of goiter across the Middle West and again an increase toward the Pacific Coast, especially in the Northern portion involving Portland, Seattle and Spokane. Another branch of this belt begins in the Eastern Pennsylvania mountains and passing Westward, takes in the beginning of the Ohio Valley and thence following the Ohio River reaches the Mississippi Valley. The cities in this group are Pittsburgh, Cincinnati, and later St. Louis.

A decade or two ago one might have stood in some shopping street in one of these cities and by ordinary inspection recognized goiter in its great prevalence in these various cities. I was in Seattle in 1920 and in one half hour in a busy shopping district counted one hundred and fifty goitrous individuals. That situation has, however, been practically eradicated. Because it was recognized that the absence of iodine was responsible for the thyroid enlargement, Dr. David Marine, then of Cleveland, proposed that small quantities of iodine be given to all persons living in those districts. This has been accomplished in various ways. In one city iodine is put into the reservoir; in one state the use of iodized table salt is said to be compulsory; in the schools of one city children receive iodine as a medicament for two weeks twice yearly; and as the medical knowledge relating to the dependence of goiter upon a lack of iodine has spread, many are using iodine voluntarily. As a result, goiter is fast disappearing as an endemic disease in the United States. However, some warning must be given that the indiscriminate use of iodine may in special cases be harmful and in those cases may convert a simple thyroid swelling into an active dangerous condition. Also, the term *goiter* used in this connection is not meant to include the conditions known as exophthalmic goiter or as toxic goiter—both of which involve many other of the glands of internal secretion and are marked, active disease processes—but simply the enlargement of the thyroid with an underactivity. Some two or three years ago I again visited Seattle, and the goiters to be seen were few and far between. The success attendant upon the general use of iodine is strikingly evident.

Later on I shall describe the change that takes place in the individual when his thyroid underactivity gives place to normality. In conclusion, it may be stated that the thyroid gland produces a substance which is absolutely necessary to the individual, in that its presence produces proper oxidation within every cell of the body. Without it, this oxidation is prevented and slowness of all bodily processes results. In later life the tissues are filled with a mucoid deposit due to this imperfect oxidation and the condition known as myxedema arises. Overproduction of thyroid secretion causes increased oxidation with all the symptoms of overactivity of all bodily processes—the heart is rapid, the temperature increased, mind unduly active, and a general loss of weight occurs.

It might be well at this point to give a short account of the picture presented by the individuals who suffer from thyroid disturbances. Because of the fact that the thyroid produces oxidation in every cell of every tissue in the body, a diminution of thyroid activity results in less activity of every tissue; therefore the hypothyroid individual, that is, one with an underactive gland, is sluggish in his physical and mental make-up. His weight increases, his secretions all diminish so that his skin remains dry, his nails become brittle, his hair falls out and he loses interest in his surroundings. There is a lowered body temperature, a slowness of the pulse rate, and a disinclination to move or work—no novelty to-day! It is difficult for him to arise early and he goes through the day in a lethargic manner. Fatigue is his constant companion.

How different the hyperthyroid individual! He is always on the move; his pulse rate is increased; his heart's action is accelerated, he is constantly in a state of mental and bodily overactivity. There is a tendency to loss of weight, a warmness of the skin, a flushing of the face and a condition of excessive perspiration. Indeed, because of the fact that his hands are moist constantly, he gets into the habit of washing them frequently and occasionally will give this habit as his most prominent symptom. With all this activity he shows usually—although this is not at all always the case—a fullness of the thyroid gland and perhaps an undue prominence of the eyeball. Restlessness is the keynote of his existence; he keeps the world moving—not always in the proper direction nor with the proper rhythm—but moving. His is no Fabian policy—he cannot wait! And nothing in the entire social world is so incompatible as the mating of a hypothyroid personality with a hyperthyroid one. The latter gets up too early in the morning, wakes up the entire household, gets every one busy and angry as a result, rushes to work and begins the same séance there. All and everything, including himself, must move. And if his mate is hypothyroidal, imagine if you can the result! A little thyroid given to the mate and a slight depressor given to the irritator, and lo, the scene changes and serenity rules. No psychological attack is necessary.

In children, however, before development is complete, the lack of thyroid is serious. As all body cells are affected, the child develops too slowly, his mind is dull, his play lacks initiative, his coördination is poor and he soon becomes deficient and more and more defective. The bony framework suffers because of late ossification, tooth formation is delayed, the genitals are underdeveloped and the hair is coarse and sparse. In the early stages thyroid medication helps him, but if too long a time elapses before this is done, the other glands become affected in turn and the situation becomes more and more complicated and more and more difficult of solution.

THE PITUITARY GLAND

Taking the next glandular element in the order of historic importance we shall discuss the pituitary gland. As you may know, this organ is situated in the base of the skull and is almost completely surrounded by a bony framework, known as the sella turcica—Turkish saddle. It is less than a half inch in length, almost a third of an inch in height and a half an inch wide—about the size of a filbert nut—and weighs about ten grains. Think of it! And it controls practically all the other glands, it controls growth, development, sexual maturity, blood pressure, pregnancy, menstruation, the water exchange of the body, many of the biochemical ingredients of the blood, and probably also mental activity. Nature, endowing it with so much power and responsibility likewise took care to protect it adequately. The bony cavity in which it is, is actually a skull itself within the real skull, and so, far from harm's way. It is surrounded on all sides by the most remarkable circular blood stream in the entire body—called the circle of Willis—so that it is almost impossible to deprive it of blood. Because it is almost hidden away, little mention is made of it by early writers for they hardly knew of its existence, or, knowing it, gave it scant courtesy on account of its size.

Galen in the second century already knew of the existence of the pituitary, however, but it was reserved for Vesalius in the sixteenth century to give it the name *Glans pituitam excipiens* because he thought that it produced the mucus which lubricated the throat (*Pituita* (Latin), meaning mucus). Because nothing else of importance could possibly be attributed to it, interest in this gland flagged for centuries. Late in the eighteenth century, curiously enough, changes were reported by Goeding of Leipzig in the pituitary gland in epilepsy. Even we moderns suspect the pituitary gland in many cases of epilepsy and many cases of improvement due to pituitary treatment are on record.

Then in 1838 there followed renewed interest in the pituitary due to a description of the development of the gland by the famous Rathke, the German anatomist. Rathke showed that the anterior part of the pituitary gland is derived from the mucous membrane of the upper pharynx and was gradually closed out from its origin by the development of the sphenoid bone of the skull which finally resulted in the almost complete inclusion of this part of the gland within the skull. This part of the pituitary gland is known as the anterior lobe. At its inclusion within the skull it joins a process coming down from the brain to which it becomes attached. This latter part derived from the brain is known as the posterior lobe. The actual division of the pituitary gland is a good deal more complicated than here appears but need not require detailed description at this time. And only two years later (1840) appears the account of an autopsy by a German physician of Würzburg, Bernhard Mohr, of a woman who had had a curious and massive obesity accompanied by mental and physical sluggishness, loss of memory and eye symptoms, and cessation of menstruation. The autopsy disclosed a tumor mass of the pituitary gland with neighborhood pressure on the adjacent cerebral parts. This was the first description of what later was to be known as the Froehlich syndrome—characterized by adiposity with sexual inadequacy. Curiously enough, this report appeared in the same medical volume that carried the first report of exophthalmic goiter by Basedow.[1]

Then came several isolated reports on acromegaly accompanied by a pituitary lesion, by Italian physicians; but it was reserved for Edwin Klebs of Königsberg to describe much more fully a case of acromegaly with both pituitary and thymus enlargements. Acromegaly, it may be explained here, is a condition of the body in which there is a progressive grossness of feature, with distortion of the skeleton, so that the spine becomes curved, the head and feet enlarged,

[1] *Wochenschrift für die Gesammte Heilkunde,* Vol. III (Berlin, 1840).

the head and face flattened and broadened and the entire picture that of the deformed court-jester. Klebs was not certain that the enlargement of these glands was not part of the general disturbance of the body and concluded that the cause must still remain obscure. It remained for the famous French neurologist, Pierre Marie, finally to describe acromegaly as a result of pituitary disease in 1886. Then in 1901, Alfred Froehlich described a case of obesity with sexual infantilism as due to the pituitary tumor which he found at autopsy. This condition was later classified by Bartels as "dystrophia-adiposo-genitalis," which it now remains. It is also known by the name of the discoverer, "Froehlich's Dystrophy."

Further studies show us that giantism is due similarly to disturbances in the activity of the pituitary gland. So that clinically, up to this time, we have thus far had described to us as a result of pituitary disturbance: growth abnormality, sexual deficiency, abnormal obesity, mental aberration, and sluggishness with somnolence. All these from a small mass of tissue of an average weight of *ten grains!*

And the story is only begun. Harvey Cushing with his associates at Harvard, Herbert Evans of California, Philip E. Smith and Carl T. Engle of Columbia, Collip of Montreal, Riddle of the Carnegie Institution, and many others in practically all the laboratories of the world have been and are now engaged on the many complex problems offered by this most perplexing gland. And as a result of their endeavors we are gradually beginning to get a faint idea of the multitudinous activities of this gland. Not only have these investigators with their associates shed much light upon the specific properties of the secretions of the pituitary but they have found out furthermore that the gland elaborates biochemical materials that control almost all the other glands in addition thereto. That is to say, there is in the anterior lobe of the pituitary a controlling substance without which the thyroid gland would deteriorate, one without which the adrenal gland would diminish its activity, one without which the parathyroid would cease functioning and finally one without which there could be no sex function. That is paramount to saying that the pituitary gland is a master gland.

To explain succinctly its specific functions: It controls growth, so that dwarfism or giantism or acromegaly are all of them its products when the growth factor indulges in vagaries. The sexual function is also one of its chief underlying charges and when it is in any way modified so that menstruation is delayed or too frequent or profuse or even absent, the pituitary anterior lobe is immediately suspect. Non-descent of the testicle in the male, or impotence, or lack of the secondary sexual characteristics may all be impugned either entirely or at least in part to the anterior pituitary. Many of the occurrences in labor, such as the contraction of the uterus preventing hemorrhage, are due to pituitary activity. Obversely, when disturbances in sexual organs occur such as disease or the removal of the testes in the young male or the ovaries in the female, the pituitary gland becomes involved and curious after effects are noticed such as abnormal growth—witness the eunuchs—a change in the voice so that it becomes high-pitched, and an abnormal growth of hair in the female, together with other pituitary effects such as increase in fat and weight, and sluggishness of mind and body. Many of these symptoms, however, can now be prevented by application of modern methods of treatment whereby substitutes for the disturbed glandular secretions are available for introduction into the body.

As before noted, the anterior lobe of the gland also has to do with the proper conversion of the fats and starches of our food. If this factor is lacking, then these food materials, instead of being utilized, simply produce additional weight of the body—obesity reigns. As the gland also controls the balance between the intake and outgo of fluids from the body, its deficiency produces too great a retention of fluid within the body and this still further increases the weight.

Another one of the newer principles discovered in the anterior lobe of the pituitary gland has been called *prolactin* by Riddle, its discoverer. This principle seems to be the one governing the production of milk. His work was done on pigeons. Both male and female birds have crop glands in the neck which secrete milk for the young squab. These crop glands develop only at maturity. But if this anterior lobe principle is injected into the very young birds many weeks before maturity, then the crop glands develop as an immediate result.

To go more intensively into these biochemical principles would merely prolong this presentation and would possibly confuse my readers. There is already enough confusion in the many paradoxical events occurring in the course of investigations by the most skilled and painstaking laboratory workers and far be it from me to add to it! But one important thing still remains to be said about the anterior pituitary. It is that when all its functions cease, a condition of cachexia results—the individual becomes weak and emaciated and his vitality is lowered to a point at which life becomes impossible. Such a condition has been brought about by Philip E. Smith of Columbia artificially in monkeys by destruction of the pituitary gland. It is known as Simmond's Disease. The posterior lobe produces, or at least contains, highly active principles, particularly, pituitrin. This biochemical product is potent in the production of blood pressure, and the maintenance of blood-sugar and therefore is of the utmost importance in shock. After surgical operation, especially in the abdomen, it is almost specific in the restoration of normal tone of the blood vessels and of the abdominal organs. It also controls the contraction of the uterus in labor. Recently it was found to consist of two separate principles—one for maintaining blood pressure, called *pitressin;* and the other controlling the uterine contraction, called *pitocin.* These have been separated from pituitrin by Kamm.

The pituitary individuals are always with us. The hypoactive ones show a mental hebetude that is quite characteristic. They acquire fat, are somewhat easygoing; they don't face their problems but go the paths of least resistance; there is no self-denial or self-abnegation. The Fat Boy in Dickens' *Pickwick Papers* is a classical example. But there is a group of hypopituitary cases that is extremely important. These cases don't get fat, but they do show markedly the trait of mental subservience. They are easily led by stronger minds. As a result and because they have no self-control they become addicts to many habits. They drink to excess or they take drugs and this latter fact makes them more and more amenable to masters who control their entire life and destiny; while under the influence of the drug they will commit any and all types of crime. The hypopituitary case cannot fix his mind properly upon his work or problems—he cannot concentrate. In youth this leads to mental deficiency. In general it may be stated that the many factors of development of stature, sex, intelligence, behavior are all held in abeyance by a deficient pituitary gland.

The other side of the picture—the hyperpituitary, is of extreme interest. The individual develops in all phases of life, he is intelligent, keen, active both mentally and physically, body well grown and well proportioned and has powers of judgment and ratiocination beyond the normal. But if the overactivity persists we get a curious let-down and a gradual picture of hypopituitarism is engrafted upon the previous state. Many so-called wonder-children belong to this group. They begin life as marvels in some activity of mind or body. In a few years, they gradually become less and less marked and then gradually decline to a normal level or even lower, and are soon lost to view. The slightly overactive pituitaric, however, is the one that leads the world, the one that bends others to his will—the one that has his plan and carries it through. Usually he pays the price through his high blood sugar and high blood pressure with a comparatively early death.

THE PARATHYROID GLANDS

We are now brought to the consideration of the next glandular element of the body—the parathyroid glands. These small bodies eluded investigators until quite recently for they are exceedingly small—but two grains in weight each. Fifty years ago they were first described by Sandström. There are four of them and they are imbedded in the thyroid gland. Curiously enough, from time to time some parathyroid tissue is also found in the thymus gland. Their function until quite recently was unknown. When the thyroid surgeons some years ago removed the entire gland in diseased states they, of course, unknowingly removed the parathyroids also. It was found out that shortly thereafter the patient, while relieved of his thyroid symptoms, began to show evidences of a condition of spasm, of muscular twitchings and then bodily convulsions occurred; and finally death took place. It was thought that meat eating produced the condition in the absence of the thyroid and as a matter of fact, meat-free diet helped the condition materially. To determine this, thyroid glands of *herbivoræ* were removed. And no convulsions occurred in them as a result of the operation. It seemed clear that meat eating was the cause. But upon closer investigation it was found that in the *herbivoræ,* the thyroid gland is distinct from the parathyroids and its removal did not include these smaller organs; therefore the conclusion was not warranted.

And so the parathyroids as a possible cause of the difficulty were studied. It was found that when they were removed in animals, even though the thyroid was left in place, the animals entered into convulsive states. A study of the blood chemistry in these animals determined the fact that their blood was very poor in calcium. And so calcium was injected into the veins of the animal whose parathyroids were removed, after which no convulsions occurred. Repetition of the experiment with various controls soon showed that the parathyroid glands determined the calcium level of the blood. It was known that the condition of body spasm called tetany was due to a lack of calcium utilization, and now the main reason of the lack was proven to lie in parathyroid underactivity. While marked diminution of calcium in the blood causes these convulsions of tetany, there are a great many states produced by a slight lessening of the calcium level below the normal which are not convulsive but which are intensely disturbing.

The action of calcium in the body is not only to supply the material out of which bone is made, but further, to act upon the muscular and nervous systems. Its presence makes the nerve currents more stable and keeps them checked and reined. As soon as it diminishes in quantity, these nerve currents become intensified and much more easily stimulated. As a result, the person with a low blood calcium perceives the most minute external stimulus which ordinarily is not appreciated. He hears the slightest sounds and is aware of the slightest environmental change. As a result he is constantly on the qui vive and hence is never in complete repose. This means that he is always at tension. He cannot relax. Therefore he sleeps poorly, is easily awakened and not sufficiently refreshed by sleep. Because of the incessant irritation of the environmental stimuli and lack of calcium control of the nerve currents, his reaction to these stimuli is quick and out of all proportion to the cause. A chance remark, a mere disapproving glance, any admonitory observation, and he is goaded to fury and gives vent to it violently. Many criminal acts are thus initiated. One of my patients, a fine intelligent boy, thus afflicted, took up a shotgun that was near him, and shot his mother because of some minor fault she was finding with him. Immediately the explosion is over, contrition enters, but too late.

Proper treatment for the utilization of calcium helps this condition immediately. This consists in giving not only calcium itself to the patient but also, in addition, parathyroid extract. In the past decade an active extract of the parathyroid gland has been isolated and prepared for general use. Both Collip and Hanson are credited with its preparation. With parathyroid overactivity, we see a disturbance produced which is highly dangerous particularly to the bony framework of the body. Because these glands increase the blood calcium this calcium must be forthcoming from some source and as the food is insufficient as a base of supplies when the glands are overactive the calcium is taken from the bones of the body. This results in a demineralization of the skeleton with cyst formation and marked weakness of the bones. As a result, spontaneous fractures result or else are produced by very slight trauma. If the parathyroid gland that is at fault can be removed surgically then the trouble is mitigated, but occasionally even after the removal of all four glands no improvement has been found. Later a large diseased parathyroid may be discovered elsewhere than in the thyroid—frequently in the thymus gland. The entire subject of the parathyroids forms one of the newer, highly important chapters, still incomplete, of the glands of internal secretion.

THE ADRENAL GLANDS

The adrenal glands next engage us. These are two in number and are found in the abdomen above the kidneys. They are composed of two distinct portions, the interior or medulla, and the shell or covering, called the cortex. It is the medulla which produces the important biochemical product "adrenalin," originally discovered simultaneously by the Japanese Takamine and Professor Abel of Johns Hopkins. This product is of the most extreme importance. It is found to increase, to at least maintain, blood pressure—to increase blood sugar, to stimulate the heart action and above all, to stimulate the sympathetic nervous system. As this nerve system controls all the involuntary activity of the body it is at once apparent that life itself depends upon the adrenal secretion. All the abdominal organs—stomach, intestines, liver, pancreas; with the organs of the thorax—heart and lungs; and the pelvic system with its genital and urinary organs are under the control of some part of this involuntary nervous system. There is some discussion as to whether adrenalin is constantly being produced and utilized or whether it is given out only in emergencies, such as shock, extreme fatigue, fright and other emotional states, as described by Cannon. One important characteristic is that it controls hemorrhage by causing contraction of the capillaries, and so may be used for such purpose in small operations. It is efficient in the smallest, almost imperceptible quantities. Abel of Johns Hopkins has shown that its presence may be detected in solution of a strength of one part in four hundred million!

The cortex of the gland furnishes one of the most recent examples of an active principle—or hormone—controlling a heretofore incurable condition known as Addison's Disease. Addison described this condition as long ago as 1849. It is characterized by bronzing of the skin and mucous membranes, progressive weakness, emaciation and finally death. No cure has been known for it. For a decade or two, however, it was surmised that the cortex of the adrenal glands was the tissue responsible for the condition and while the active principle had not been isolated it was referred to as "hormone X." Finally, however, it was given to two investigators almost simultaneously to discover and produce it. Hartmann of Buffalo and Swingle of Princeton both succeeded in isolating the principle—now called *cortin,* from the adrenal cortex, some five years ago. This active agent when injected into sufferers from Addison's Disease causes an almost immediate response. From being moribund, they almost immediately begin to sit up and take notice, acquire an appetite and improve in all their symptoms. As this result is fairly temporary, however, cortin must be given daily or even oftener. It is a very expensive preparation and beyond the means of many sufferers, and so much time and thought are being given to prepare a more simple and cheap method of treatment.

From this short synopsis of the work done by the adrenal glands, one can readily see that without them, life would be impossible. One extremely interesting fact is that the cortex of the glands is composed of the same kind of cellular element as goes to the structure of the genital organs—notably, the ovary. And as a result, disturbance of the cortex, such as inflammation or tumor, produces a change in the secondary sexual characteristics. In the female particularly, there is an abnormal growth of hair—even to the formation of a mustache or beard—and finally the entire body becomes covered with coarse hair. At the same time, menstruation ceases, and with these events a marked personality change enters, masculinity being its keynote. It is curious to note that practically all the glandular elements of the body have many functions to perform, not only to maintain biochemical balances but to maintain as well external appearances and psychic reactions. Probably all three are correlated functions of an underlying principle and the combinations of all these underlying glandular principles make up the complexity of the individual—no wonder no two human beings are alike!

THE GONADS

We are now led almost directly to the consideration of the genital glands. As stated earlier in this discussion, from time immemorial these glands were the object of the greatest solicitude for they were recognized as the basic tissue for the continuation of the race. And when it was apparent that they were not functioning normally, all means were taken to correct the disturbance. And almost invariably these means were to utilize the sex tissue of animals as correctives. These tissues were prepared in all possible ways: decoctions, broths, tinctures, extracts, and even the raw material was used as food, and curiously enough with frequently favorable results. This one glandular treatment of a glandular deficiency has come down to us through the ages and was utilized by all peoples. It remained for a one-time professor of Harvard, Dr. Brown-Sequard toward the end of the nineteenth century to place this treatment on a more or less rational basis. He prepared a solution of testicular material from animals and injected this into himself. He had gradually been becoming tired and jaded with oncoming age and believed he could thus fortify himself against too rapid senility. The results apparently justified all his theories for his mental and physical stamina returned and renewed vigor asserted itself. This date of his report to the French medical world, May 31, 1889, is now regarded as the birth of modern endocrinology. Much water has gone over the dam since then and the genital organs, or gonads as they are termed, have become the center of the recent intensive investigation into the glandular system. To go into details of these investigations would exhaust the reader's interest and patience but in so far as results are concerned these are epochal.

In the first place, two American physicians, Allan and Doisy, discovered almost a decade ago, 1929, the active principle of one of the component tissues of the ovary—the follicular tissue. This active principle named *folliculin* or *theelin* is that which prepares the living membrane of the uterus for the reception of the ovum after it is fertilized. In a general way it stimulates the entire genital tract. Should the ovum not have been fertilized, then this living membrane is shed in the next menstrual flow. After the ovum is discharged from the ovary where it has been developed, a small blood clot remains in the site of rupture. This blood clot becomes organized and then is known, because of its yellowing color, as the corpus luteum, which has an effect to prevent the shedding of the uterine membrane. That is to say it is in a measure antagonistic to theelin (from the Greek θῆλυς, "female," and *"in"*). When the ovum, however, is fertilized, then the activity of the corpus luteum is prolonged for practically the entire length of time necessary to the complete development of the ovum into the fetus and finally into the child, ready to be delivered into the world. And this activity of the corpus luteum prevents the menstrual flow and shedding of the uterine membrane during the entire gestational period, and therefore conserves the race. From it, the ovarian principle "progestin" is prepared. When this ceases to function at full term, then the uterus empties itself and a newcomer is ushered in. While this all seems to be an activity of the ovary, yet it has been found that the anterior lobe of the pituitary gland is sponsor for the initiation of much, if not all of the ovary's activity.

Without the presence of this pituitary anterior lobe gonadal hormone, these events would not occur. Now comes a highly interesting corollary to the whole matter. Should the ovum become fertilized and there is no further use for ovarian activity during pregnancy, what becomes of the secretions, theelin and that gonadal principle of the anterior lobe of the pituitary gland which are now not needed? They are excreted largely in the urine. Therefore, if we examined the urine of pregnant women we ought to find evidence of such gonadal extracts in it. And they ought to produce their effects on ovaries in other individuals if they were injected into them. And this is exactly what we find they do. Therefore, if we examine the urine of a woman in whom we wish to diagnose the presence or not of pregnancy and find that it contains these ovary stimulating properties, then pregnancy is practically positively assured. How is the test made? Injections of the urine are made into immature rats and if within a few days these rats show in their ovaries the results of stimulation, seen in the enlargement and maturity of the glands and the bleeding points of the corpora lutea, then the test for pregnancy is positive. This test can be made in the first few weeks of the suspected pregnancy and is almost completely satisfactory. The test is known as the Aschheim-Zondek test. A few years ago the diagnosis for pregnancy could not be positively made before the third month. It has always been a most interesting subject for debate as to the time when the rupture of the ovum from the ovary takes place for it is at this time or very shortly thereafter that fertilization must take place. Most recently this time has been partially fixed as about midway between two menstrual periods. This represents the most promising time for the fertilization of the ovum. The remainder of the month is known among women as the "safe period."

When it comes to the male gonads we have a somewhat different and simpler arrangement. There are two types of tissue, one being the sperm and the other known as the interstitial tissue producing an active principle which controls the secondary sexual characteristics of the male. We need not dwell upon the activity of the spermatozoa—they take all too good care of themselves! But the interstitial tissue needs some explanation. It is this tissue which is assumed to be at the basis of man's virility and youth, and it is this tissue to which he directs himself for the delights of rejuvenation. All possible methods for extracting and utilizing its active principles are in vogue and none up to the present time has given much promise. The so-called Steinach operation which engaged so much attention in recent years, is an attempt to increase the activity of the interstitial tissue by irritating it through tying off the duct through which the spermatozoa leave the testicle. This results in retention of the sperm cells within the gland causing irritation and congestion with resulting stimulation of the interstitial cells. This causes presumably increased vigor and mentality and generally a rejuvenation. Some cases have apparently shown improvement in these respects, even to the restoration of youthful hair coloring. Nothing is said, however, of the danger of overburdening old arteries through increasing vigor and activity. One hears much less nowadays of this much advertised operative procedure than of yore.

Interesting is the experimental work on the gonads by which through transplantation of female ovaries into males with removal of the testes, and the transplantation of testes into females with removal of the ovaries, the complete transformation into the other sex of these operated animals can be brought about.

Thus Oscar Riddle speaks of a case in which a fowl, originally a mother and laying eggs, became later a father with the production of male germ cells. And there are several not thoroughly authenticated cases of like character that have been reported as occurring in humans. Even the possibility of parthogenesis in humans has been shown to exist. What determines the sex of an individual originally is as yet not known but in all probability this is fixed at the moment of fertilization.

PANCREAS AND INSULIN

A short description must now of necessity be given of the gland, the pancreas (Greek: πᾶς, all, plus κρέας, meat) which is not ductless but has an internal secretion. This organ, situated just below the stomach, has a duct through which it supplies the intestinal contents with several of the digestive juices that have to do with the conversion of starches, fats and proteins. While experimenting on dogs deprived of their pancreas, an attendant in the laboratory of Minkowski noticed that large swarms of flies were attracted to the urine passed by these dogs and not to that of the other control animals. This led to a chemical examination of this urine which was found filled with sugar. Thus the effect of the pancreas as a whole on sugar control was immediately suspected and later established. By methods of elimination it was soon proven that the part of the pancreas concerned in this sugar metabolism was the groups of cells known as the Islands of Langerhans.

Many investigators then set themselves to the task of deriving from these cells their active principle. It was finally accomplished in the laboratory of Professor McLeod of the University of Toronto by Dr. F. G. Banting and C. H. Best in 1921. They were assisted in the work and partially directed by Dr. McLeod and Dr. J. B. Collip. This active principle, called *insulin,* was the result of their labors. It is supererogatory to tell you of the importance of this discovery. It not only helped thousands of human beings that had been suffering from the condition known as diabetes from an early and certain death (in which disease there is an inability to oxidize and utilize sugar), but it immediately placed the entire subject of internal glandular disease upon a high physiological plane. It quieted many of the scoffers and antagonists of this "quasi-medical" science and led them into the fold. It has been said that the original paper published by the Toronto group was refused at first by almost all medical journals as too sensational for belief. The Nobel Prize was awarded to them nevertheless and their names will go down in medical history as among the greatest benefactors of mankind. It must be remembered, however, that insulin is not a "cure" for diabetes, but simply a substitutive treatment for the lack of the proper pancreative principle.

THE THYMUS

Finally, we reach in our march the thymus gland. Actually this gland ought to be considered first in our course for it is preëminently the gland that is active during our early years. It is situated within the thorax above the heart and in close relationship to it. It weighs about one ounce at birth and gradually increases in size to the tenth year, after which it gradually involutes. At times, small rests may be found during life but so far as we now know its activity practically ceases at puberty. Its recognition as a gland has been and still is widely disputed, for experiments in feeding, in removal and by injection have often had paradoxical—not to say negative—results. Its removal in dogs has been shown to produce disturbances in skeleton growth, resembling rickets, so that the legs became bowed and the dogs stunted. To confirm this result, similar experiments were made a decade ago at Johns Hopkins, and almost completely negative results were produced—no change in the skeleton resulted! As for feeding, Gudernatsch fed thymus to tadpoles and produced marked increase in growth so that he had actual giant tadpoles—but they did not develop into frogs. So that the conclusion was drawn that the thymus produced growth but hindered development. Later on, an Italian, Soli, showed that fowl with the thymus removed produced eggs without a shell. If these same fowl were fed with thymus gland the egg again had the shell. Riddle showed similar results in doves. From these experiments it became evident that the thymus gland had to do with lime or calcium metabolism and therefore the idea that it produced growth again arose. In the last three years Rowntree, with an active principle of the thymus prepared by Hanson succeeded in accelerating the growth of white rats in a surprising way when given to successive generations. And in addition, and in contradiction to previous investigators these rats also developed much more rapidly. Their eyes opened earlier, and their genitals matured in half the normal time.

Interesting to note was the fact that the pituitary gland in these rats showed an increase in the size and number of the sex cells, the basophiles, as well as the growth cells, the acidophiles. The thymus evidently produced a pituitary activity. However, these experiments of Rowntree as yet lack complete confirmation by others. When we consider the thymus gland in man and its apparent effect clinically on him we witness partial confirmation of animal experimentation. Thus in children with large thymus glands, growth in height is usually abnormal, but development in them is retarded. They remain children in many respects longer than the average, and they show these childhood traits in many ways. Their skin is velvety and smooth—peaches and cream in character. Their hair is soft and silky, no mustache hairs make their appearance until very late, if at all—and the body hair is almost absent. The genitals remain small and undeveloped and sometimes take on the character of the other sex.

However, intelligence is not usually in abeyance and later, when proper compensations in the glandular system arise, these children develop into adults of usually superior quality although their arrival at complete development is much later than normal. But during their childhood, and even later, if proper compensation does not occur, they suffer from the lack of proper development in many important organs. The heart and blood vessels are too small, the pituitary and adrenal glands are too small and they are inefficient. These factors make for great fatigability. The sex glands are undeveloped. And because the body growth is so great and its proportions incorrect, their joints are loose and they are subject to all manner of dislocations—so-called double-joints. Because the joints of the arch of the foot are so pliable, flatfoot results; and because of the laxness of the joint between spine and pelvis, backache on undue exercise is produced; and so we have an individual that in many ways is incapable of competing with his fellows. This changes his psychological aspect and he becomes shy, cannot meet his problems, and therefore becomes a mere follower and never an aggressor. There is no actual proof that the thymus overactivity produces such individuals, but these individuals do possess enlarged thymus glands and the involution of the gland is delayed.

In early life the thymus gland may be so large that it impedes proper breathing, and if it is drawn into the upper entrance into the chest, it may so interfere with the nerves and blood vessels there situated that death may ensue rapidly. This is the so-called mors-thymica. Children with large thymus glands may have all the appearance of perfect health. Upon sudden undue exertion, they become cyanotic and collapse.

It has been found, however, that because of the small and thin blood vessels in this condition, such exertion may produce a rupture in one of the blood vessels in some important vital organ, such as the brain, or the suprarenal gland or even in the artery supplying the heart, and the sudden death is then attributable to this cause rather than to the actual size of the thymus gland. Between the children that die this early death and the mature, thoroughly compensated adult that began life with a large thymus, there are hosts of individuals that only partially compensate and carry their troubles, due to this lack of complete maturity, throughout life. They are always tired, cannot concentrate well, have fugacious pains involving the back, or the foot, or the heart; have low blood pressure, don't react well to cold or exercise, and in general have such a wrong mental attitude to life that they are dubbed neurasthenic or hysterical or are even found among the psychically disturbed. Many of our shell-shocked cases in the war belong to this group.

Then there are individuals that have too small a thymus gland and while the diagnosis is difficult, it has been shown that these cases are quite the reverse of those just cited. They mature early, but remain small in stature and are of the old-young type. Mustache and beard and early general maturity occur and they show a curious mental attitude of precocity without the basis of knowledge or experience. Because of these characteristics they prove a bane to society.

GENERAL

There are several other important organs that have so-called internal secretions but because of the highly technical character of the biochemistry involved or because of the failure to prove the presence of one as yet unrecognized active principle—they are omitted in this paper. These are the pineal gland, the liver, the intestinal mucosa, the spleen.

Finally we may note that the span of human life may be divided logically into three great epochs: the first, from birth to maturity; the second, from maturity to the prime; and lastly, from the prime through senescence to death. During each of these periods, because the goal of each is different from the others, a different equipment is necessary. During the first period, when maturity is the objective, all the glandular elements that make for growth and accretion are in the ascendant. When maturity is attained, and all man's powers are to be utilized in the procreation of his kind and in the struggle for existence in sharp competition, then the glandular activity of the pituitary, the thyroid, the adrenals, and the gonads is called forth in the highest degree. When this second period has reached its acme, no further biological reason exists for man's further survival and he gradually, with his glandular mechanism, fades into the composite picture of the human race.

([1])